Essential Clinical Signs

M J Jamieson MRCP (UK)
Lecturer, Department of Medicine
and Therapeutics, University of
Aberdeen

H M A Towler MRCP (UK) FRCSE
Lecturer, Department of
Ophthalmology, University of
Aberdeen

K P Duguid FRPS
Director, Department of Medical
Illustration, University of Aberdeen

J C Petrie FRCP FRCPE
Professor, Department of Medicine
and Therapeutics, University of
Aberdeen

K C McHardy MRCP (UK)
Lecturer, Department of Medicine
and Therapeutics, University of
Aberdeen

Gwen Chessell MEd
Coordinator, Medical Learning
Resources Group, University of
Aberdeen

T M MacDonald BSc MRCP (UK)
Lecturer, Department of Medicine
and Therapeutics, University of
Aberdeen

Churchill Livingstone

EDINBURGH LONDON MELBOURNE AND NEW YORK 1990

CHURCHILL LIVINGSTONE
Medical Division of Longman Group UK
Limited

Distributed in the United States of America
by Churchill Livingstone Inc.,
1560 Broadway, New York, N.Y. 10036, and
by associated companies, branches and
representatives throughout the world.

First published 1990

ISBN 0-443-04206-3

**British Library Cataloguing in Publication
Data**

Jamieson, M. J.
    Essential clinical signs.
    1. Man. Diseases. Physical signs
    I. Title
    616.07′2

**Library of Congress Cataloging in
Publication Data**

Essential clinical signs / M.J. Jamieson . . . [et. al.].
    p.   cm.
    1. Symptomatology—Atlases.   2. Diagnosis—Atlases.   I. Jamieson,
M. J., MRCP (UK)
    [DNLM: 1. Diagnosis—atlases.   WB 17 E78]
RC69.E87   1990
616.07′5—dc20

Produced by Longman Group (FE) Ltd
Printed in Hong Kong

This illustrated vocabulary of medical signs in internal medicine will be of interest to students in all branches of health care. The 402 images have been selected by experienced medical teachers and illustrators. The aim has been to show the common or classical clinical signs which students, often junior, are expected to recognise. Clearly a student who may have read about the sign but has not yet seen it is unlikely to recognise and report it. Once seen, never forgotten!

The illustrations have been chosen from the extensive slide library of the Department of Medical Illustration of the University of Aberdeen. The collection should be of special value for self-learning. It poses questions in the reader's mind and inevitably will stimulate the reader to further background reading.

In order to make the book more accessible to an international market, each of the captions has been translated into French, German and Spanish in the special International Glossary.

The authors have enjoyed preparing the collection which has been loosely organised along the broad lines of a physical examination. In most of the captions one, sometimes two, signs have been highlighted. We would have liked to include even more essential signs, and gradations of signs, but have restricted the examples to provide a book within a realistic price range. We hope that readers will share our enjoyment of successfully recognising the signs!

MJJ
KCMcH
HMAT
GC
KPD
TMMacD
Aberdeen, 1990   JCP

Acknowledgements

We would like to acknowledge the cooperation of the following colleagues in contributing material for this book:

Dr N Bruce Bennett; Miss F M Bennett; Dr P D Bewsher; Mr C T Blaiklock; Dr J Broom; Dr P W Brunt; Mr P B Clarke; Dr Gaynor Cole; Dr Audrey A Dawson; Professor A S Douglas; Dr J G Douglas; Dr A W Downie; Dr C J Eastmond; Dr Neil Edward; Mr J Engeset; Mr O M Fenton; Professor J V Forrester; Dr J A R Friend; Mr W H H Garvie; Mr Frank Green; Professor R L Himsworth; Dr A W Hutcheon; Mr C Hutchinson; Dr T A Jeffers; Dr A W Johnston; Mr R Keenan; Dr A C F Kenmure; Dr J S Legge; Dr R A Main; Mr K L G Mills; Dr N A G Mowat; Mr I F K Muir; Dr Lilian E Murchison; Mr W J Newlands; Dr D W M Pearson; Dr J Petersen; Dr J M Rawles; Mr P K Ray; Mr C R W Rayner; Dr D M Reid; Dr J A N Rennie; Professor D S Short; Dr C C Smith; Dr L Stankler; Professor J Stowers; Dr J Webster; Dr Marion I White; Dr M J Williams; Mr G G Youngson.

We wish also to thank the patients who gave permission for their photographs to be reproduced here; general practices, the Primary Care Division and the Medical Records Department of Grampian Health Board for their help in tracing patients; and the staff of the Department of Medical Illustration of the University of Aberdeen.

Contents

Head and neck

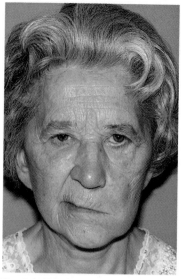

Fig. 1 Left facial palsy—lower motor neurone

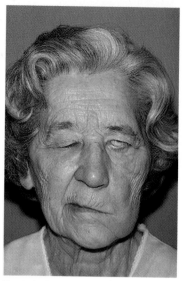

Fig. 2 Left facial palsy—closing eyes

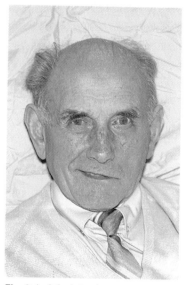

Fig. 3 Left facial palsy—upper motor neurone

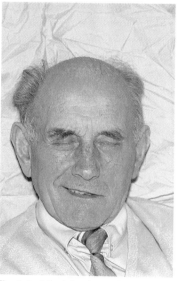

Fig. 4 Left facial palsy—closing eyes

Fig. 5 Jaundice

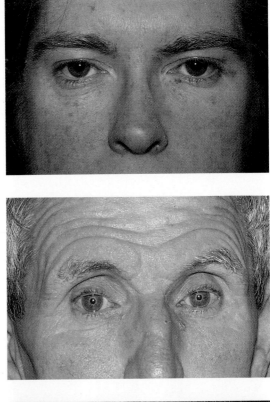

Fig. 6 Jaundice

Fig. 7 Jaundice

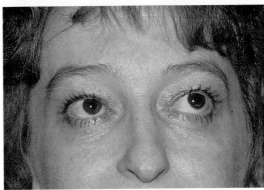

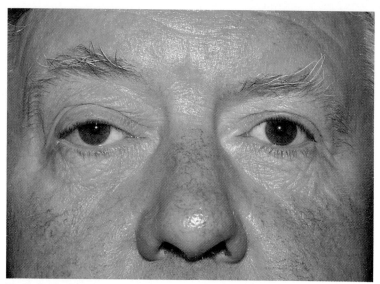

Fig. 8 Telangiectasia

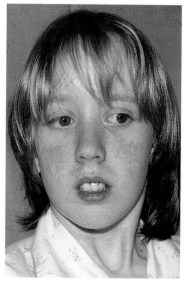

Fig. 9 Butterfly rash

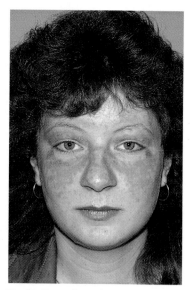

Fig. 10 Butterfly rash

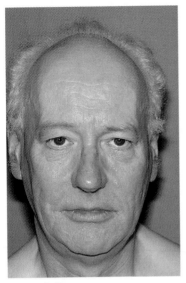

Fig. 11 Pallor

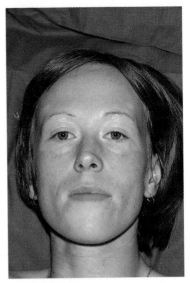

Fig. 12 Vitiligo

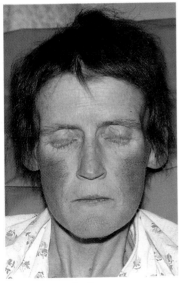

Fig. 13 Malar flush

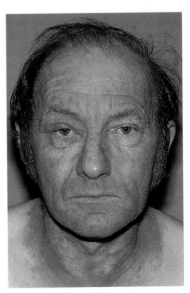

Fig. 14 Photosensitive rash

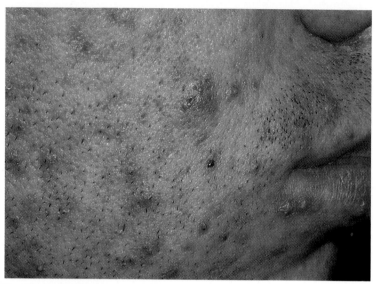

Fig. 15 Acne vulgaris

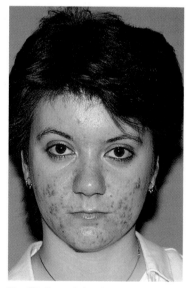

Fig. 16 Acne vulgaris

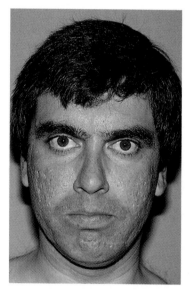

Fig. 17 Acne scarring

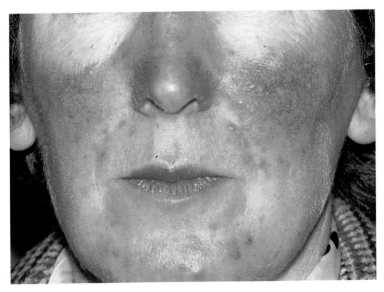

Fig. 18 Rosacea

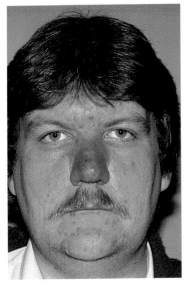

Fig. 19 Rosacea

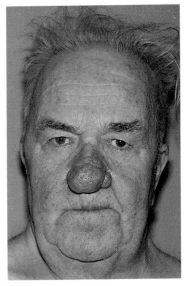

Fig. 20 Rhinophyma

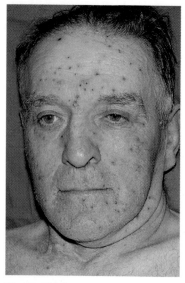

Fig. 21 Chickenpox

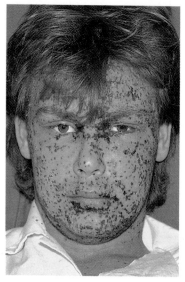

Fig. 22 Kaposi's varicelliform eruption

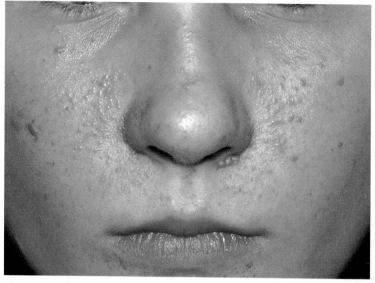

Fig. 23 Adenoma sebaceum

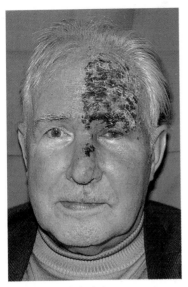

Fig. 24 Ophthalmic herpes zoster

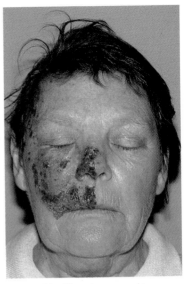

Fig. 25 Maxillary herpes zoster

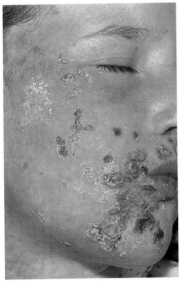

Fig. 26 Mandibular herpes zoster

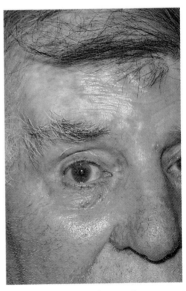

Fig. 27 Post-herpetic scarring

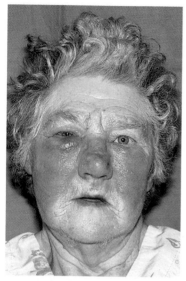

Fig. 28 Facial cellulitis

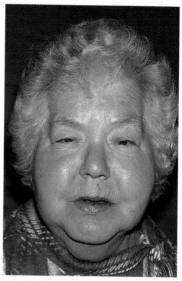

Fig. 29 Facial swelling

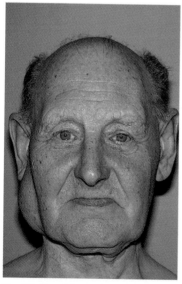

Fig. 30 Parotid swelling

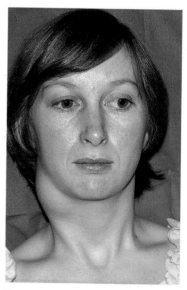

Fig. 31 Branchial cyst

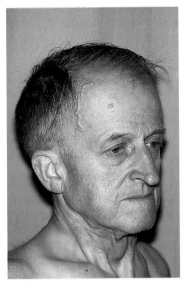

Fig. 32 Pagetic skull

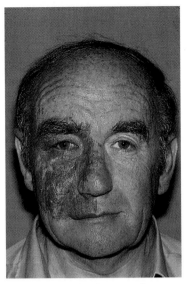

Fig. 33 Cavernous haemangioma (port-wine stain)

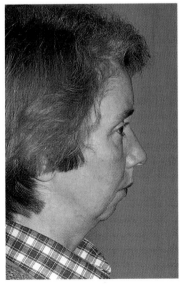

Fig. 34 Micrognathia

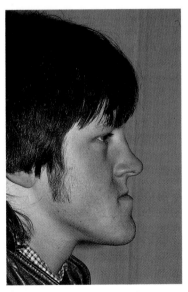

Fig. 35 Prognathia

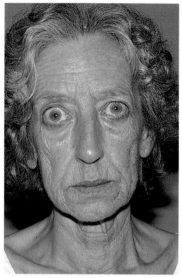

Fig. 36 Thyrotoxicosis

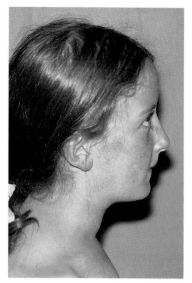

Fig. 37 Goitre

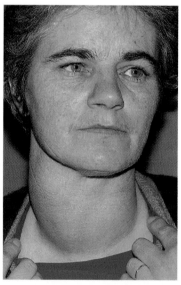

Fig. 38 Goitre

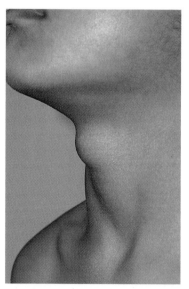

Fig. 39 Thyroglossal cyst

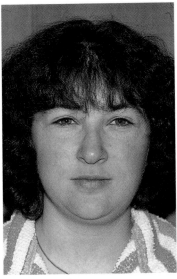

Fig. 40 Hypothyroidism

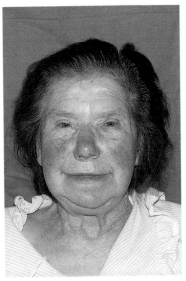

Fig. 41 Hypothyroidism

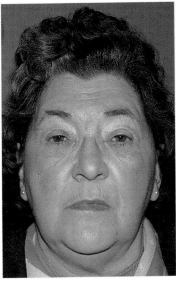

Fig. 42 Hypothyroidism—
untreated

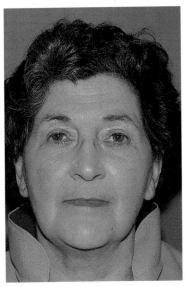

Fig. 43 Hypothyroidism—treated

13

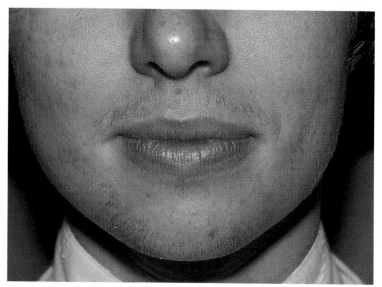

Fig. 44 Hirsutism

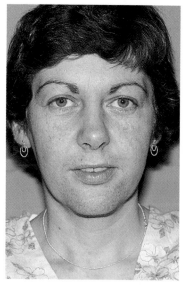

Fig. 45 Hirsutism

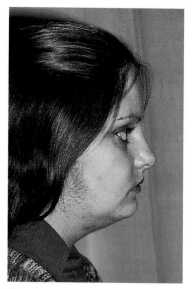

Fig. 46 Hirsutism

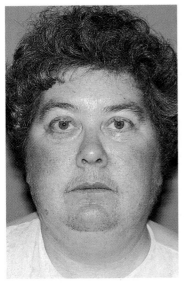

Fig. 47 Cushing's syndrome—spontaneous

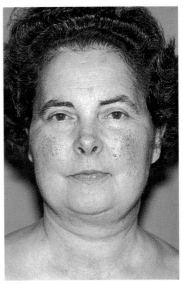

Fig. 48 Cushing's syndrome—iatrogenous

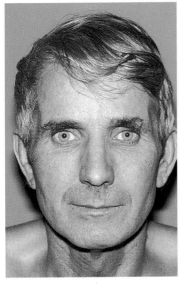

Fig. 49 Addisonian pigmentation

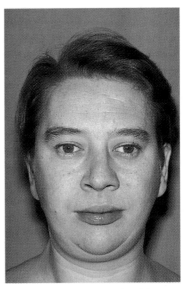

Fig. 50 Hypopituitarism (male)

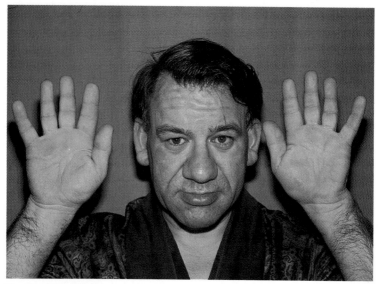

Fig. 51 Acromegaly

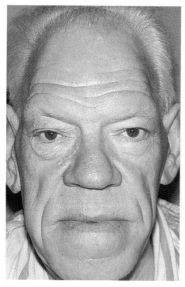

Fig. 52 Acromegaly

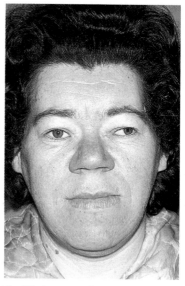

Fig. 53 Acromegaly

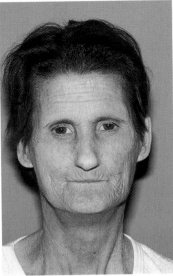

Fig. 54 Progressive systemic sclerosis

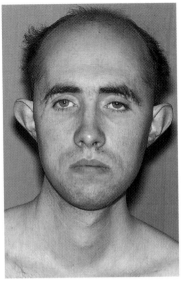

Fig. 55 Myotonic dystrophy

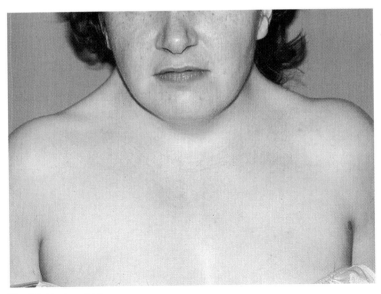

Fig. 56 Neck webbing

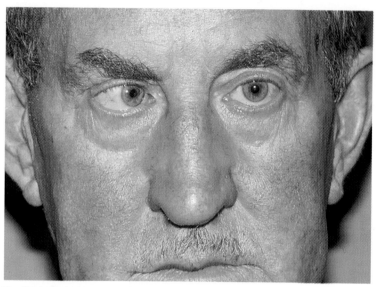

Fig. 57 Left sixth-nerve palsy—looking left

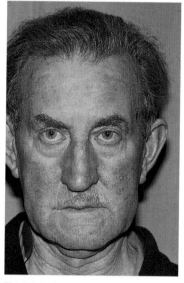

Fig. 58 Left sixth-nerve palsy—
looking ahead

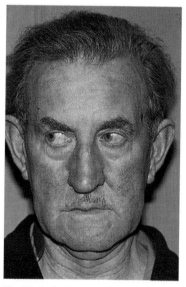

Fig. 59 Left sixth-nerve palsy—
looking right

18

Fig. 60 Left third-nerve palsy—complete ptosis

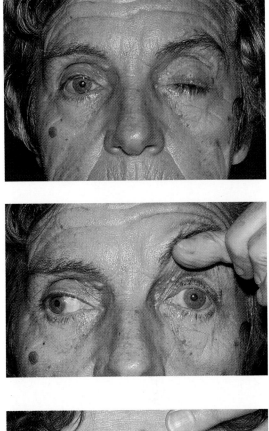

Fig. 61 Left third-nerve palsy—looking right

Fig. 62 Left third-nerve palsy—pupillary dilatation

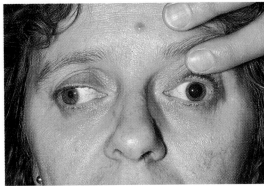

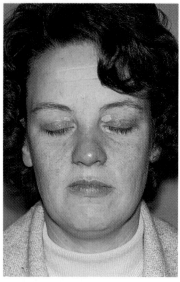

Fig. 63 Xanthelasmata

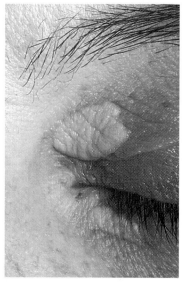

Fig. 64 Xanthelasmata

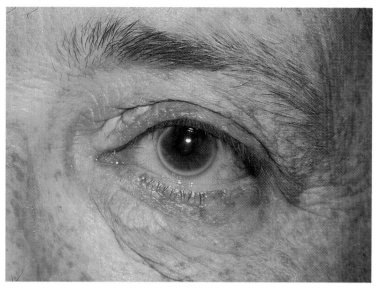

Fig. 65 Xanthelasmata and corneal arcus

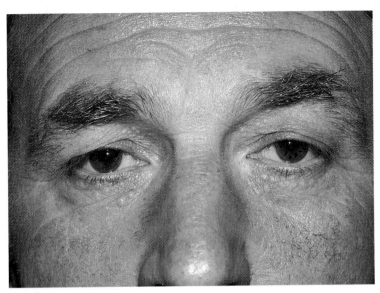

Fig. 66 Xanthelasmata

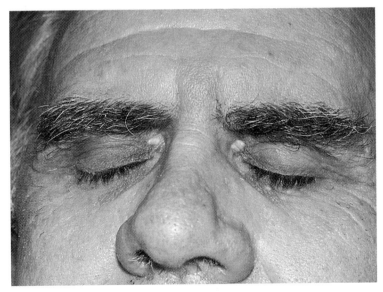

Fig. 67 Xanthelasmata

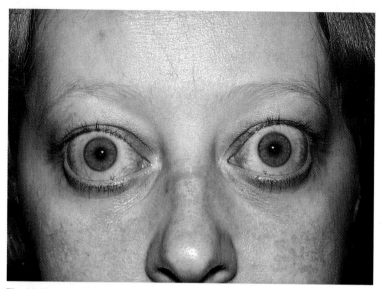

Fig. 68 Dysthyroid eye disease: upper and lower lid retraction

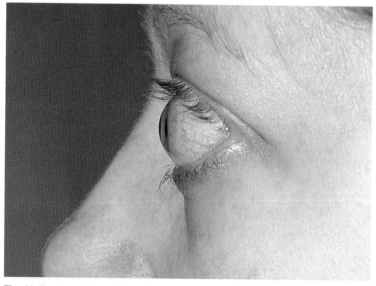

Fig. 69 Dysthyroid eye disease: proptosis

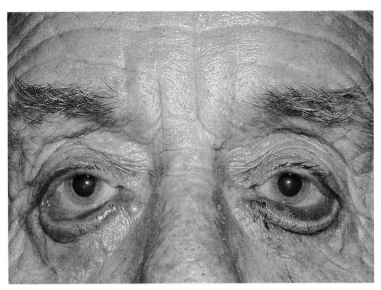

Fig. 70 Bilateral ectropion

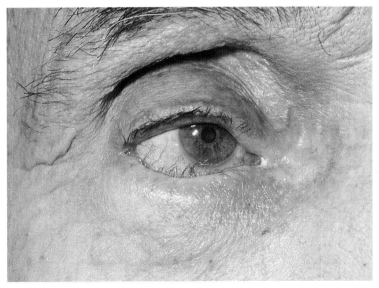

Fig. 71 Entropion

23

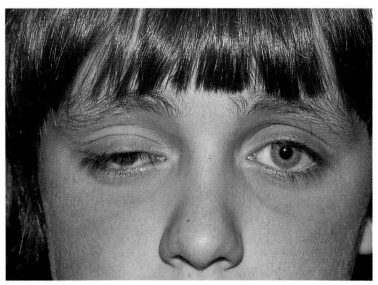

Fig. 72 Ptosis—congenital

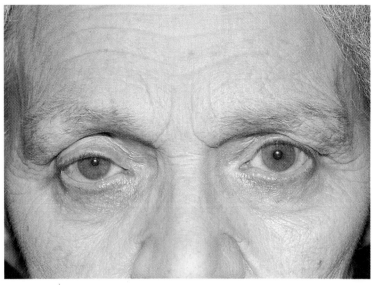

Fig. 73 Ptosis—acquired: Horner's syndrome

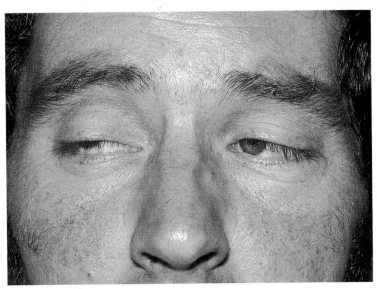

Fig. 74 Myasthenia gravis—bilateral ptosis

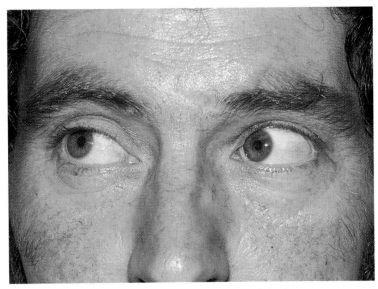

Fig. 75 Myasthenia gravis—after anticholinesterase injection

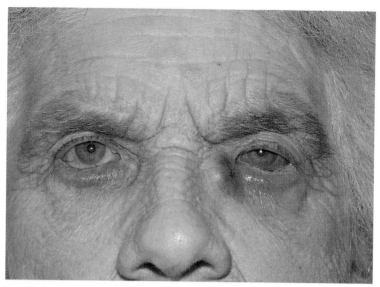

Fig. 76 Dacryocystitis

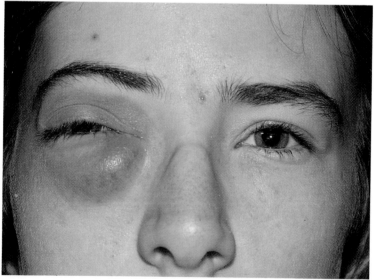

Fig. 77 Orbital cellulitis

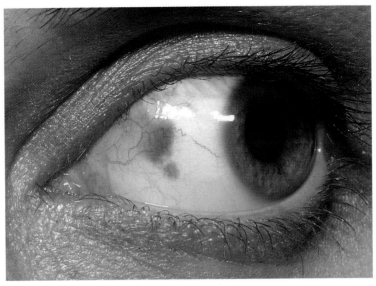

Fig. 78 Subconjunctival haemorrhage—spontaneous

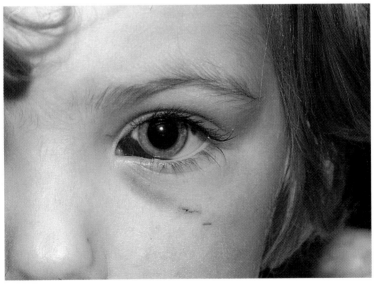

Fig. 79 Subconjunctival haemorrhage—traumatic

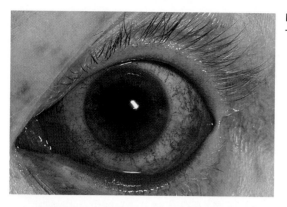

Fig. 80 Conjunctivitis
—limbal pallor

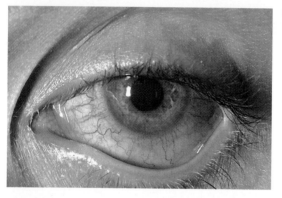

Fig. 81 Iritis—limbal
injection

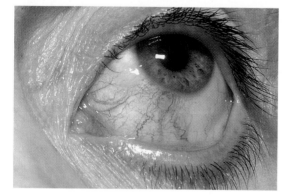

Fig. 82 Episcleritis

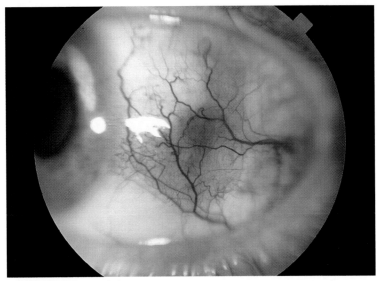

Fig. 83 Scleritis—nodular

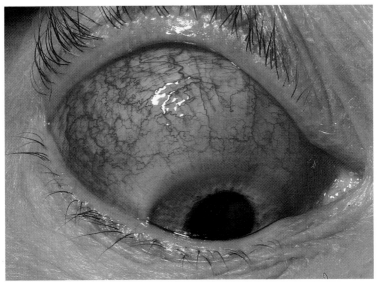

Fig. 84 Scleritis—diffuse

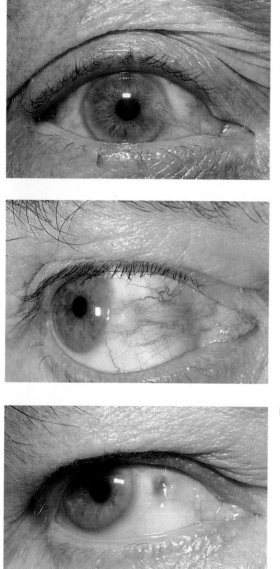

Fig. 85 Pterygium

Fig. 86 Pinguecula

Fig. 87 Scleromalacia

30

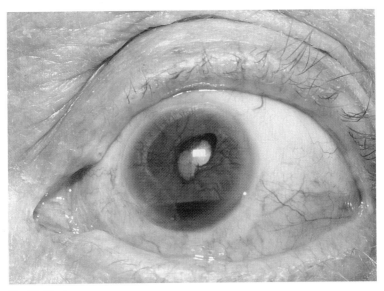

Fig. 88 Hyphaema

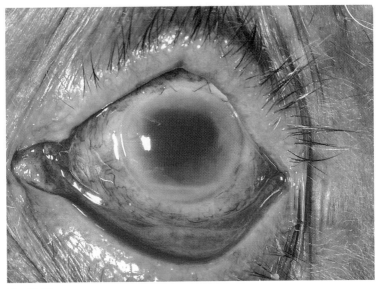

Fig. 89 Hypopyon

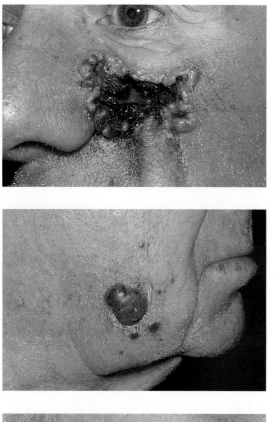

Fig. 90 Basal cell carcinoma (rodent ulcer)

Fig. 91 Malignant melanoma

Fig. 92 Lentigo maligna

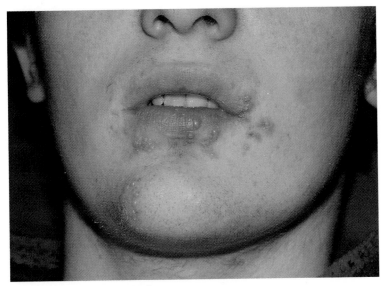

Fig. 93 Herpes simplex labialis

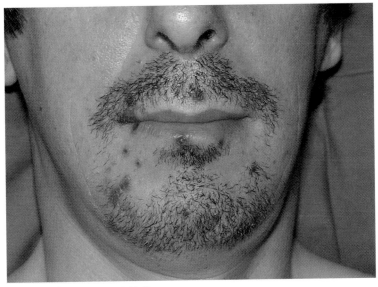

Fig. 94 Herpes simplex labialis

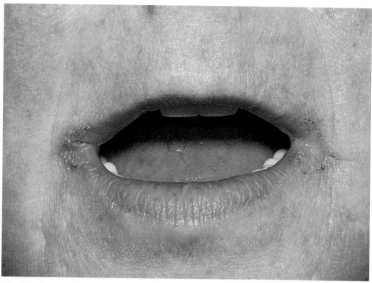

Fig. 95 Angular stomatitis

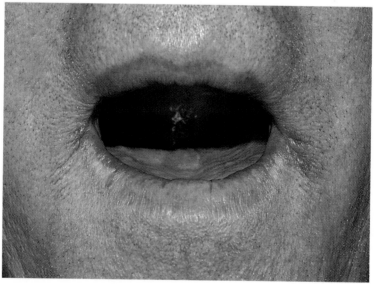

Fig. 96 Angular stomatitis

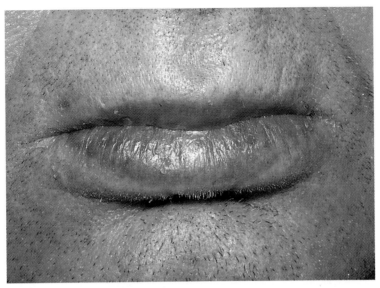

Fig. 97 Central cyanosis

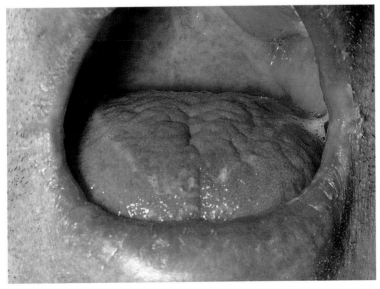

Fig. 98 Central cyanosis

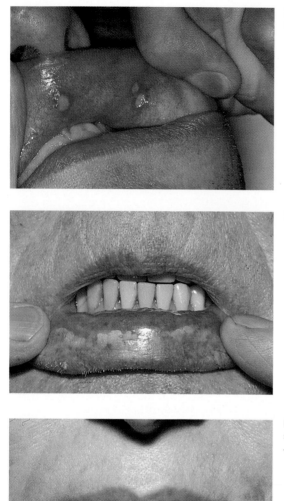

Fig. 99 Buccal ulceration

Fig. 100 Leukoplakia

Fig. 101 Pigmented spots: Peutz-Jegher's syndrome

Fig. 102 Dental caries

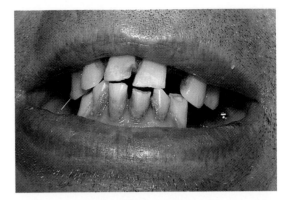

Fig. 103 Tetracycline staining

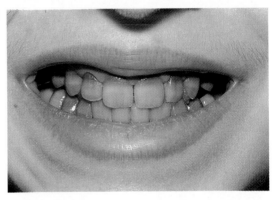

Fig. 104 Gum hyperplasia

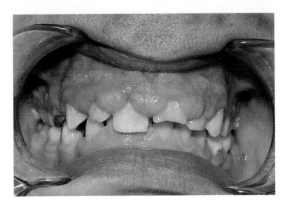

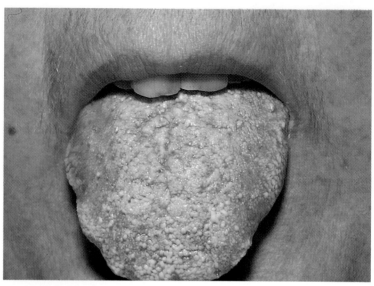

Fig. 105 Candidiasis

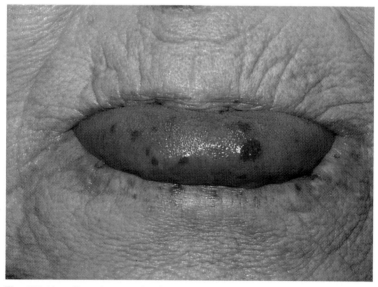

Fig. 106 Hereditary haemorrhagic telangiectasia

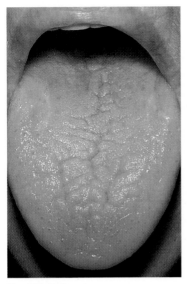

Fig. 107 Pallor

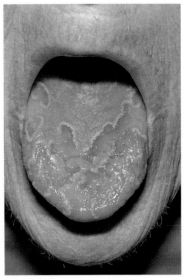

Fig. 108 Geographic tongue

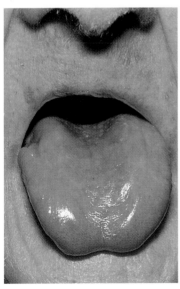

Fig. 109 Atrophic glossitis

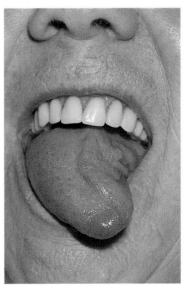

Fig. 110 Left twelfth-nerve palsy

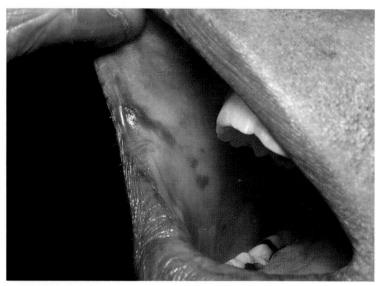

Fig. 111 Buccal pigmentation

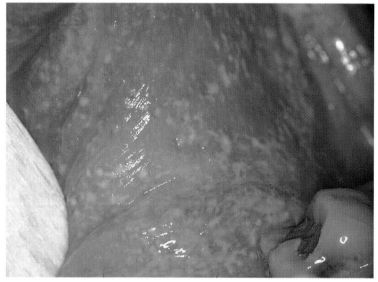

Fig. 112 Lichen planus

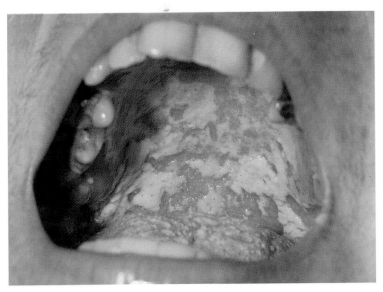

Fig. 113 Candidiasis

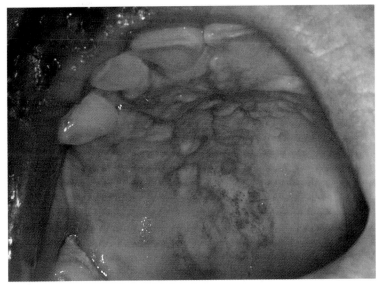

Fig. 114 Herpes zoster

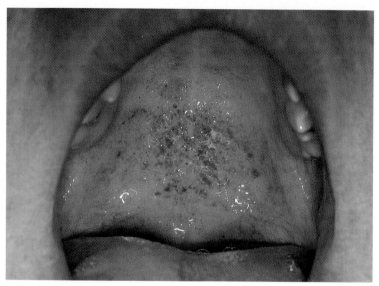

Fig. 115 Palatal petechiae

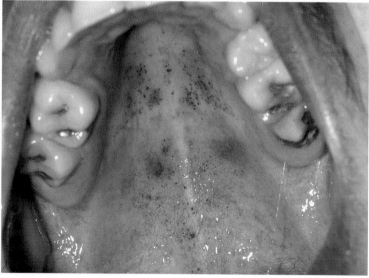

Fig. 116 Palatal petechiae

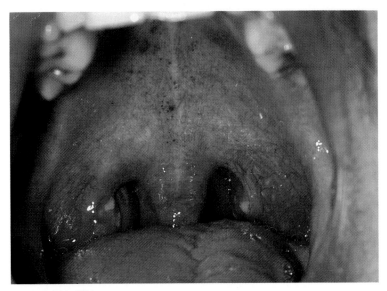

Fig. 117 Tonsillitis

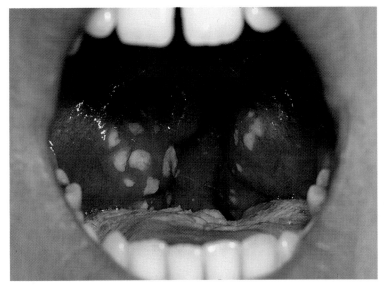

Fig. 118 Tonsillitis

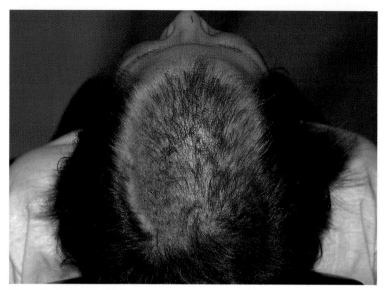

Fig. 119 Alopecia—diffuse

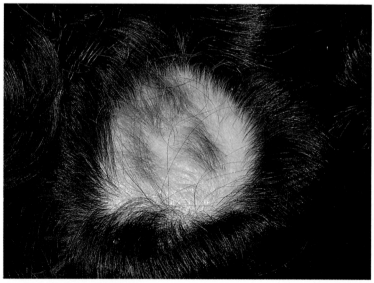

Fig. 120 Alopecia—patchy

44

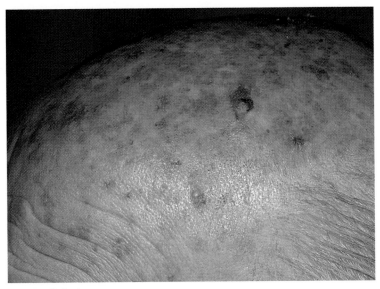

Fig. 121 Solar keratoses

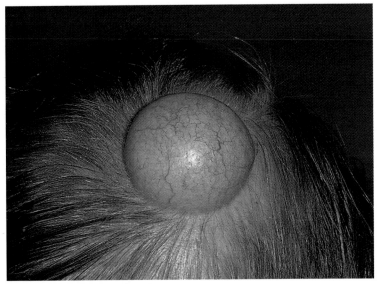

Fig. 122 Sebaceous cyst (wen)

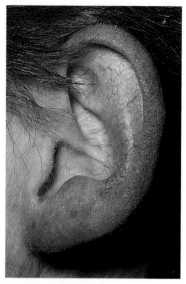

Fig. 123 Peripheral cyanosis

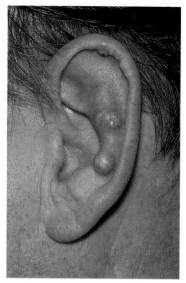

Fig. 124 Gouty tophi

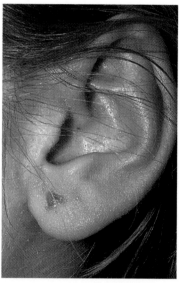

Fig. 125 Contact dermatitis

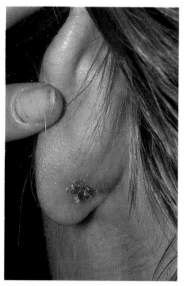

Fig. 126 Contact dermatitis

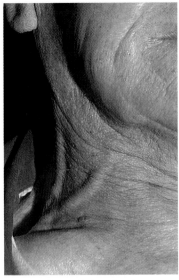

Fig. 127 Distended neck veins

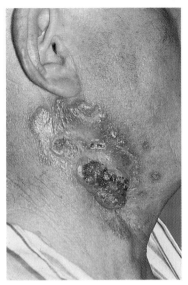

Fig. 128 Scrofula

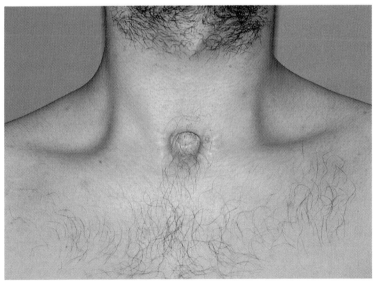

Fig. 129 Tracheostomy scar

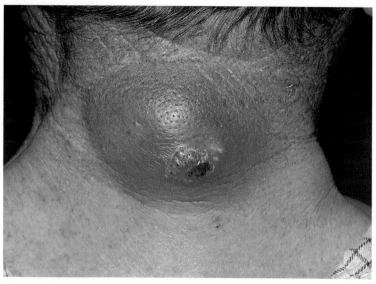

Fig. 130 Carbuncle

Hands, arms and axillae

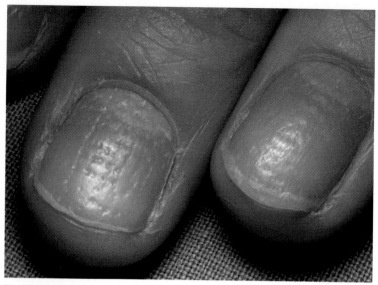

Fig. 131 Nail pitting

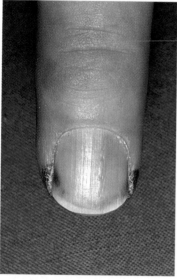

Fig. 132 Nail fold infarcts

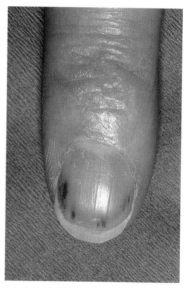

Fig. 133 Splinter haemorrhages

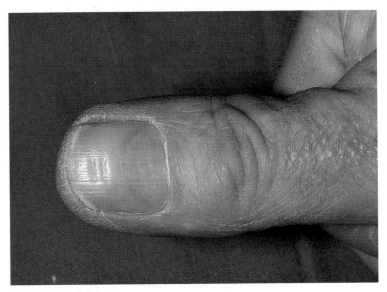

Fig. 134 Beau's lines

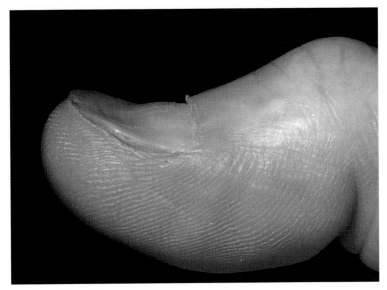

Fig. 135 Koilonychia

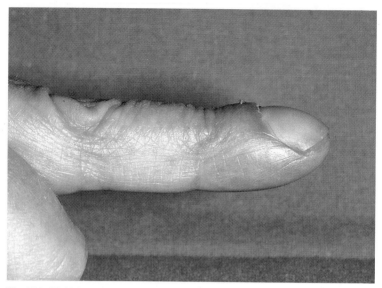

Fig. 136 Clubbing—increased longitudinal curvature

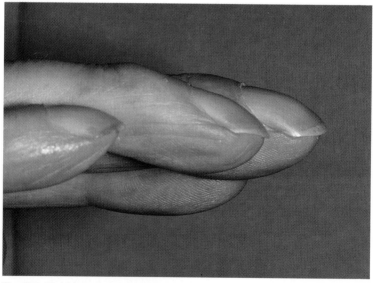

Fig. 137 Clubbing—loss of nailbed angle

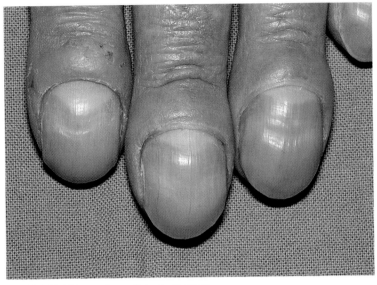

Fig. 138 Clubbing—drumstick appearance

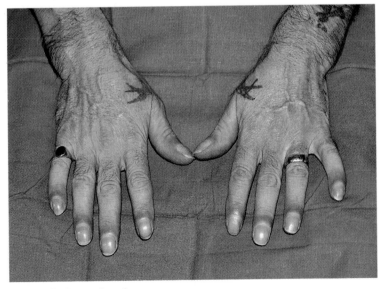

Fig. 139 Periungual erythema

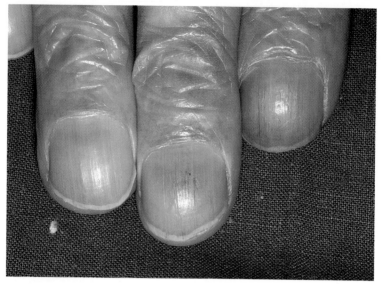

Fig. 140 Tar (nicotine) staining

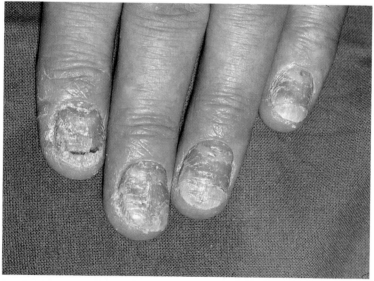

Fig. 141 Nail dystrophy

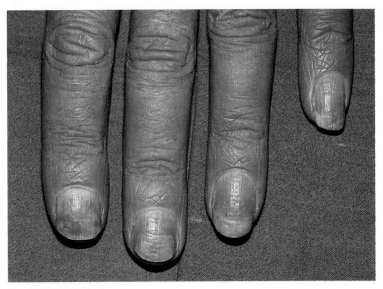

Fig. 142 Onycholysis

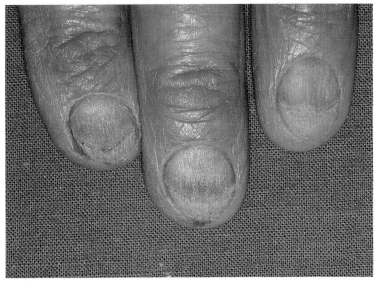

Fig. 143 Onycholysis

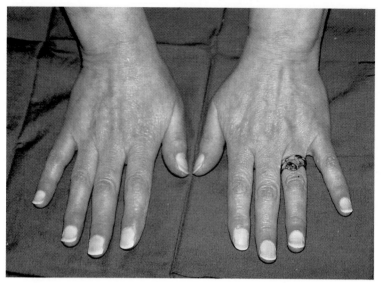

Fig. 144 Leukonychia

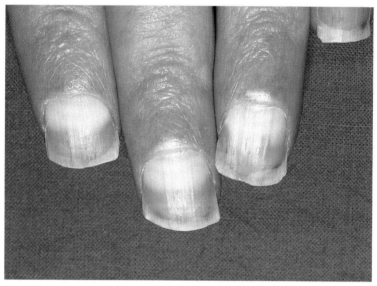

Fig. 145 Leukonychia

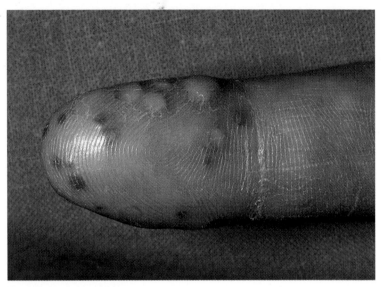

Fig. 146 Herpetic whitlows

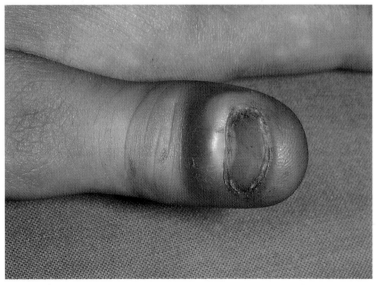

Fig. 147 Paronychia

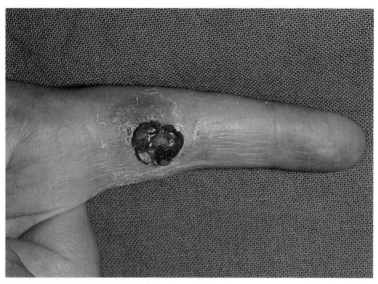

Fig. 148 Pyogenic granuloma

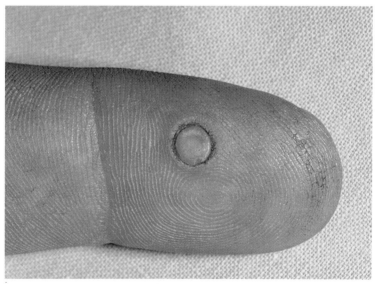

Fig. 149 Inclusion dermoid

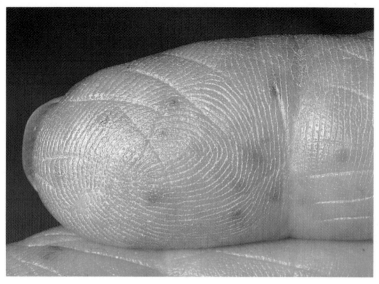

Fig. 150 Hereditary haemorrhagic telangiectasia

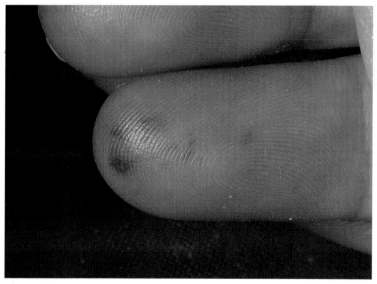

Fig. 151 Osler's nodes

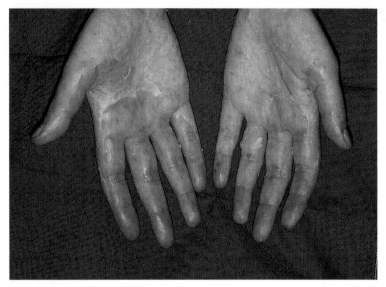

Fig. 152 Desquamation

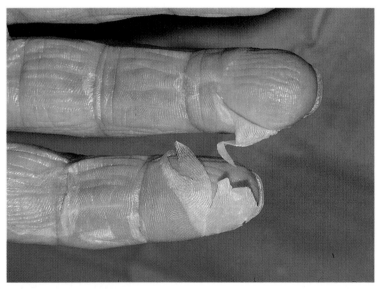

Fig. 153 Desquamation

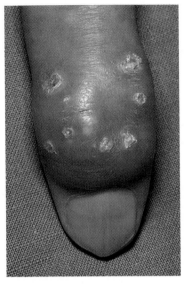

Fig. 154 Gouty tophi

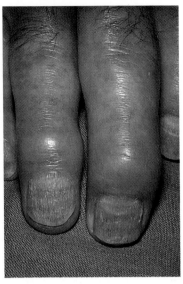

Fig. 155 Psoriatic arthropathy and nail dystrophy

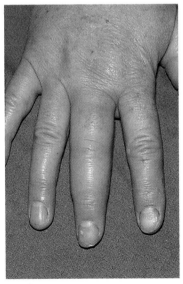

Fig. 156 Dactylitis—psoriatic

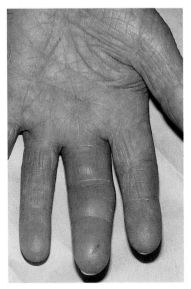

Fig. 157 Dactylitis—infective

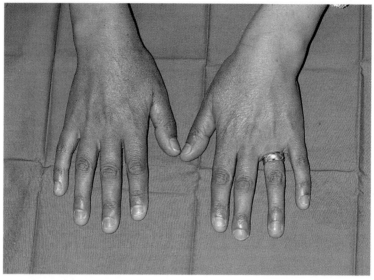

Fig. 158 Melanin pigmentation

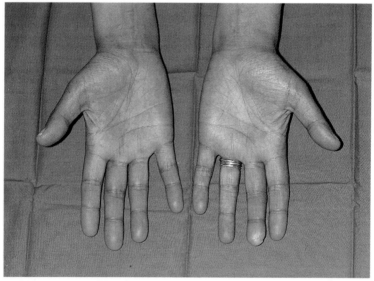

Fig. 159 Melanin pigmentation

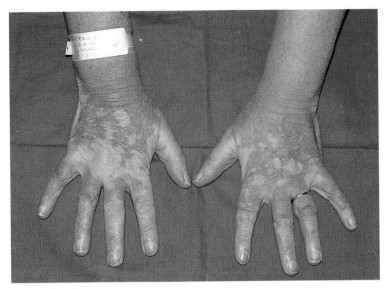

Fig. 160 Vitiligo

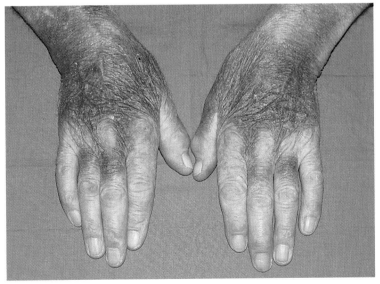

Fig. 161 Steroid purpura

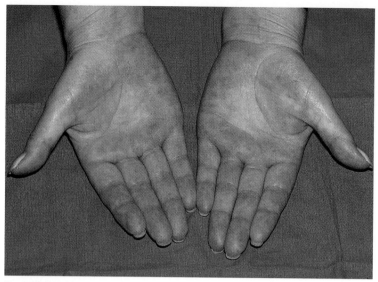

Fig. 162 Palmar erythema

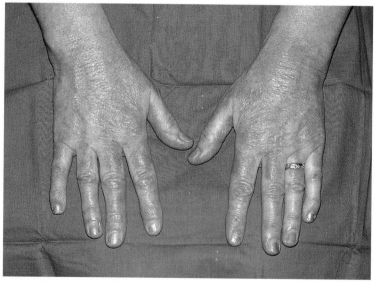

Fig. 163 Dermatomyositis

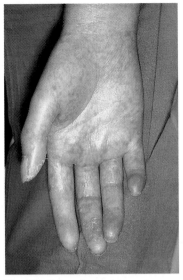

Fig. 164 Scleroderma

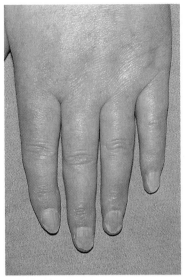

Fig. 165 Scleroderma

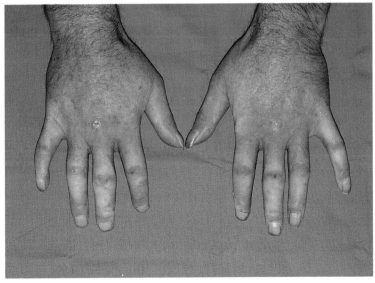

Fig. 166 Scleroderma

65

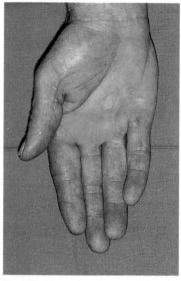

Fig. 167 Dupuytren's contracture

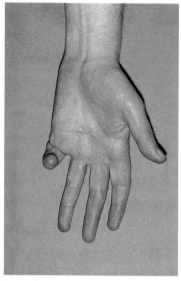

Fig. 168 Dupuytren's contracture

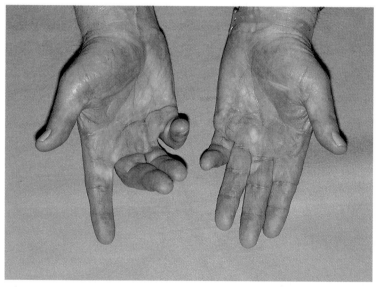

Fig. 169 Dupuytren's contracture

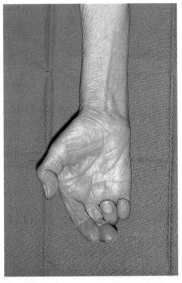

Fig. 170 Ulnar nerve palsy—claw hand

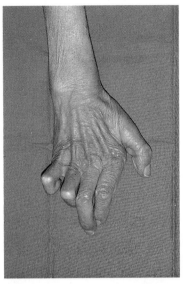

Fig. 171 Ulnar nerve palsy—claw hand

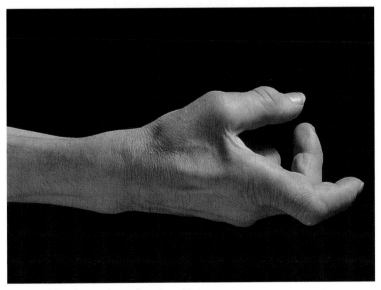

Fig. 172 Muscle wasting—first dorsal interosseus

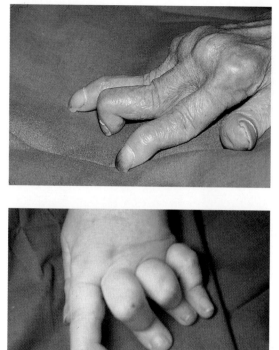

Fig. 173 Rheumatoid arthritis—swan-neck deformities

Fig. 174 Rheumatoid arthritis— boutonnière deformities

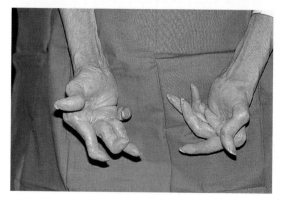

Fig. 175 Rheumatoid arthritis—swan-neck and Z-thumb deformities

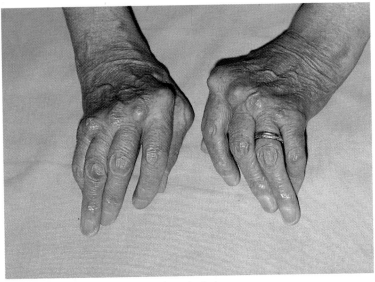

Fig. 176 Rheumatoid arthritis—ulnar deviation

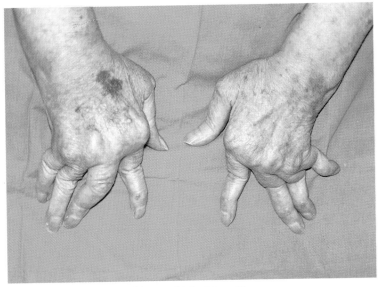

Fig. 177 Rheumatoid arthritis—multiple deformities

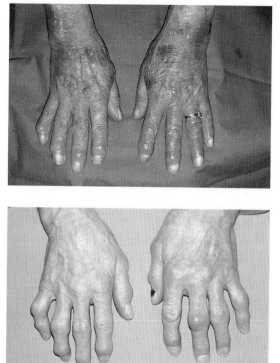

Fig. 178 Heberden's nodes

Fig. 179 Heberden's and Bouchard's nodes

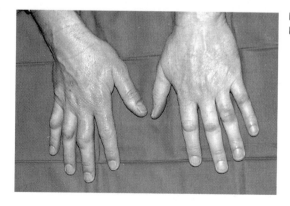

Fig. 180 Garrod's pads

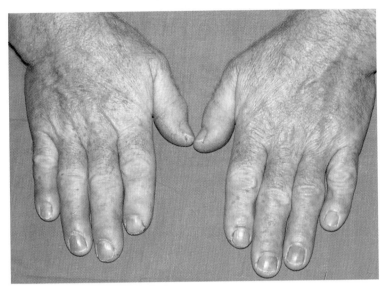

Fig. 181 Acromegaly

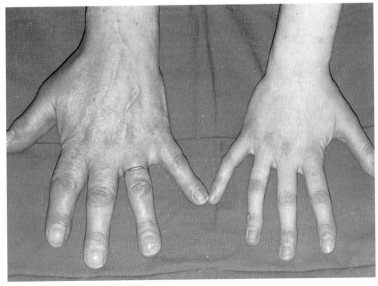

Fig. 182 Acromegalic and normal hands

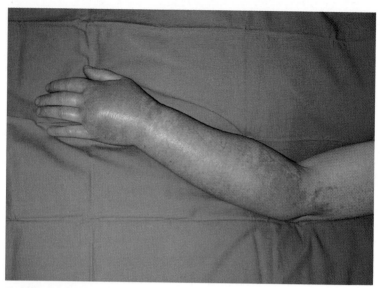

Fig. 183 Cellulitis

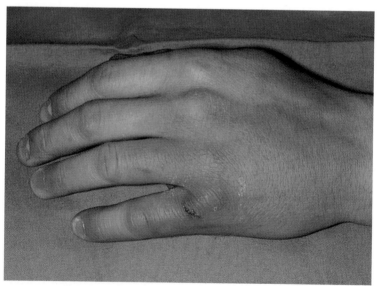

Fig. 184 Cellulitis

Fig. 185 Track marks ('mainlining')

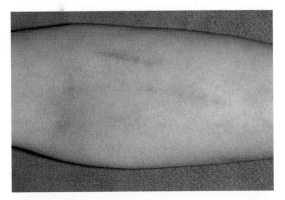

Fig. 186 Lymphangitis

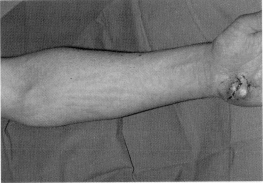

Fig. 187 Lymphangitis

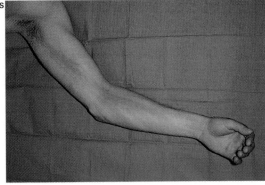

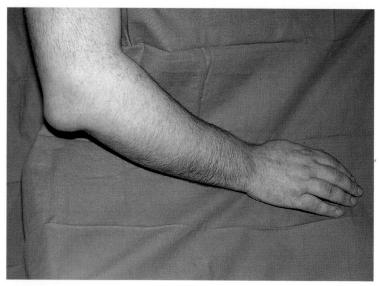

Fig. 188 Olecranon bursa

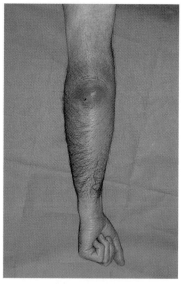

Fig. 189 Olecranon bursitis

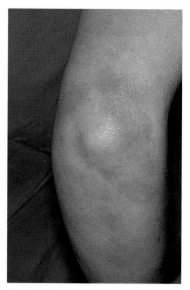

Fig. 190 Erythema nodosum

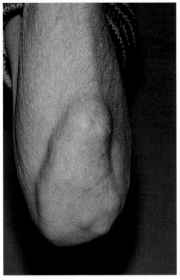

Fig. 191 Rheumatoid nodules

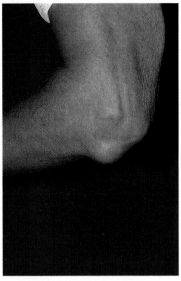

Fig. 192 Rheumatoid nodules

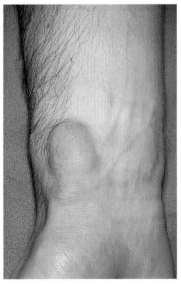

Fig. 193 Ganglion

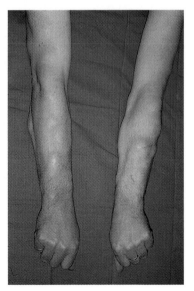

Fig. 194 Lipomata

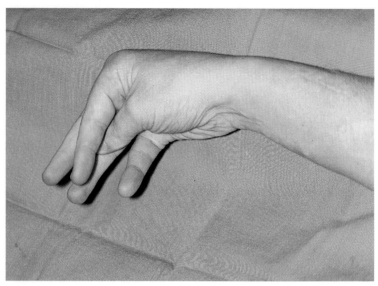

Fig. 195 Main d'accoucheur

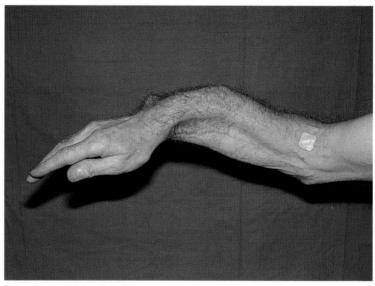

Fig. 196 Pagetic forearm

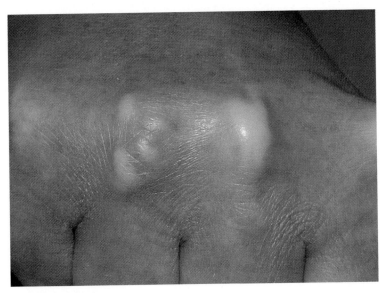

Fig. 197 Xanthomata

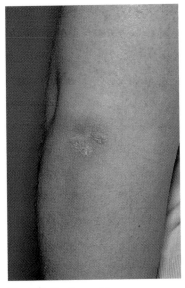

Fig. 198 Xanthomata

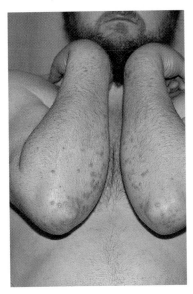

Fig. 199 Xanthomata

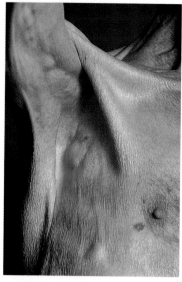

Fig. 200 Lymphadenopathy

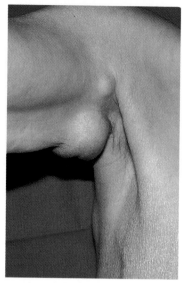

Fig. 201 Lymphadenopathy

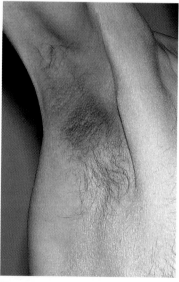

Fig. 202 Acanthosis nigricans

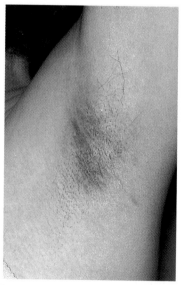

Fig. 203 Pseudoacanthosis

Chest, abdomen and genitalia

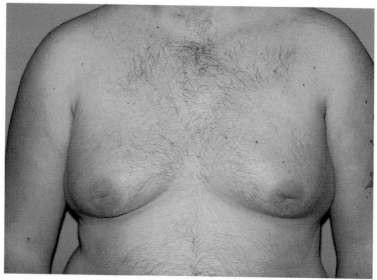

Fig. 204 Gynaecomastia

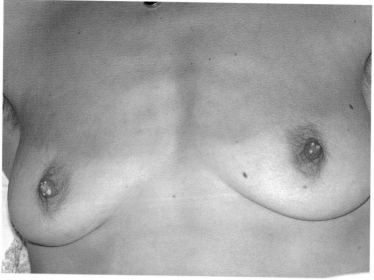

Fig. 205 Galactorrhoea

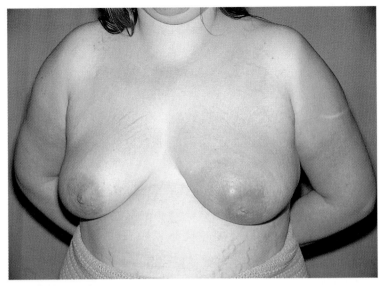

Fig. 206 Breast abscess

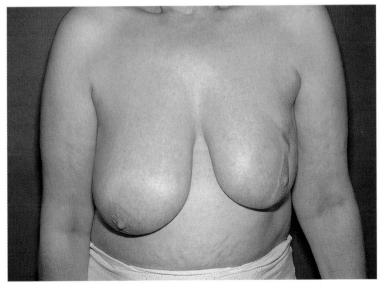

Fig. 207 Breast carcinoma

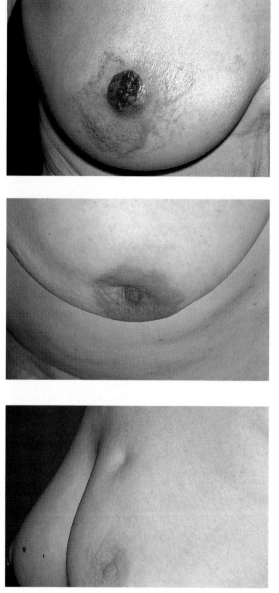

Fig. 208 Paget's disease of nipple

Fig. 209 Breast carcinoma—nipple retraction

Fig. 210 Breast carcinoma—skin tethering

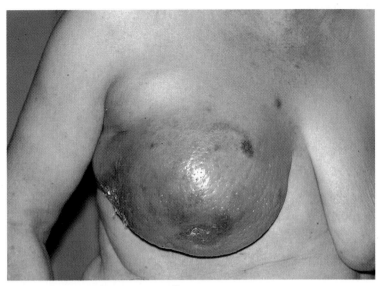

Fig. 211 Breast carcinoma—peau d'orange

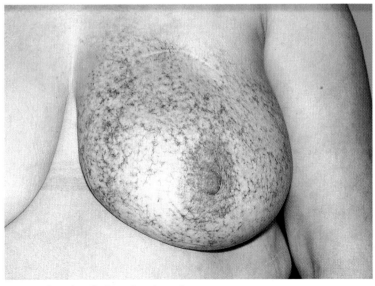

Fig. 212 Post-irradiation telangiectasia

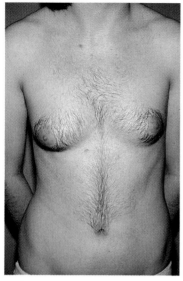

Fig. 213 Hirsute female

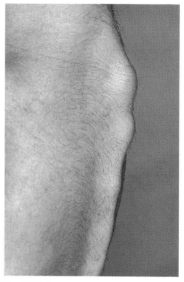

Fig. 214 Lanugo: anorexia nervosa

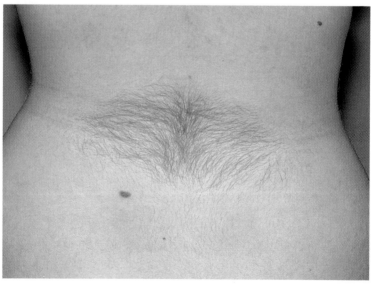

Fig. 215 Spina bifida occulta

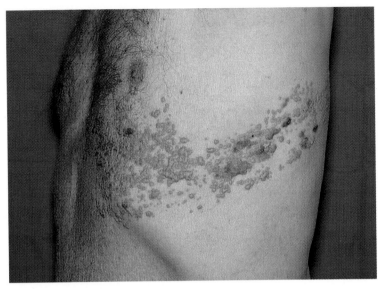

Fig. 216 Herpes zoster

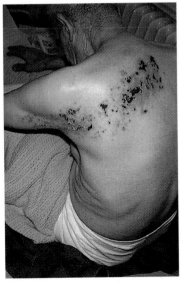

Fig. 217 Herpes zoster

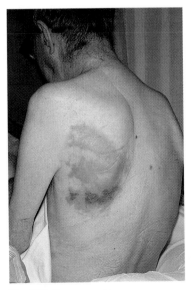

Fig. 218 Herpes zoster

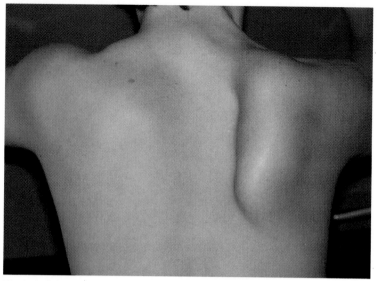

Fig. 219 Winged scapula

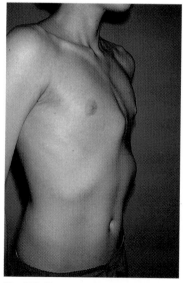

Fig. 220 Pectus carinatum

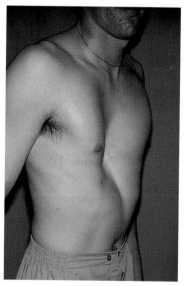

Fig. 221 Pectus excavatum

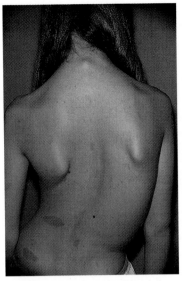

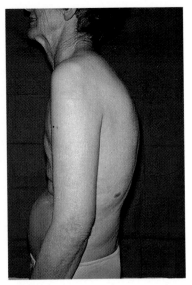

Fig. 222 Scoliosis and café au lait patches

Fig. 223 Kyphosis

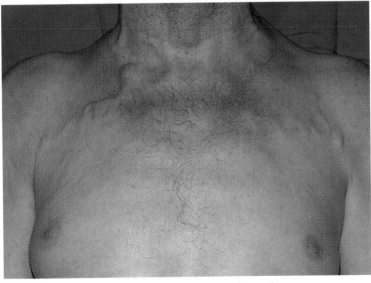

Fig. 224 Venous distension: superior vena cava obstruction

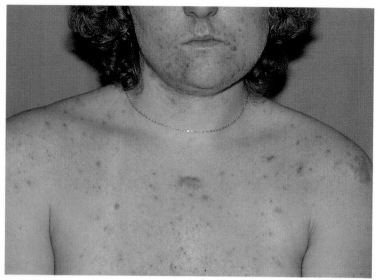

Fig. 225 Acne vulgaris

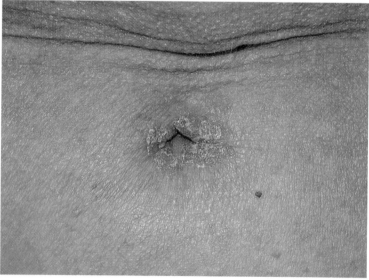

Fig. 226 Umbilical psoriasis

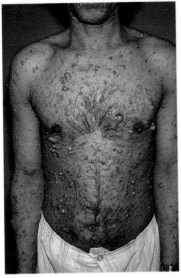

Fig. 227 Neurofibromatosis

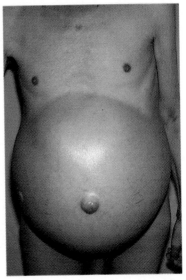

Fig. 228 Abdominal distension with everted umbilicus

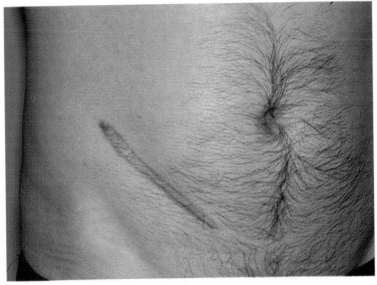

Fig. 229 Pigmented scar: Addison's disease

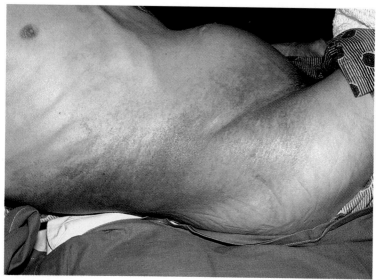

Fig. 230 Gray-Turner's sign

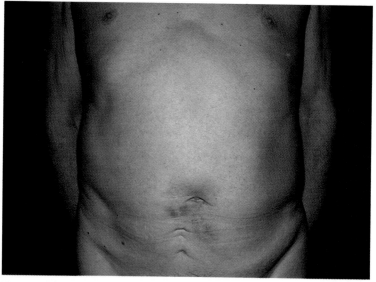

Fig. 231 Cullen's sign

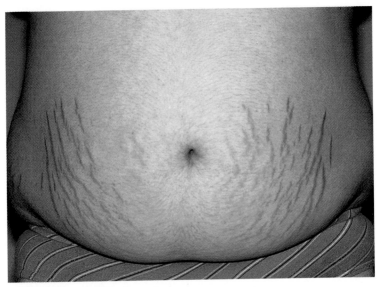

Fig. 232 Striae: Cushing's syndrome

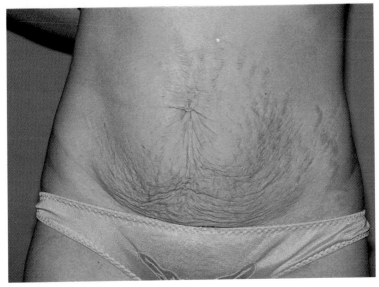

Fig. 233 Striae gravidarum

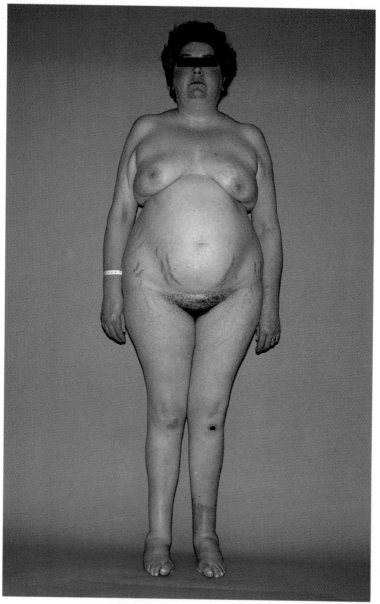

Fig. 234 Cushing's syndrome

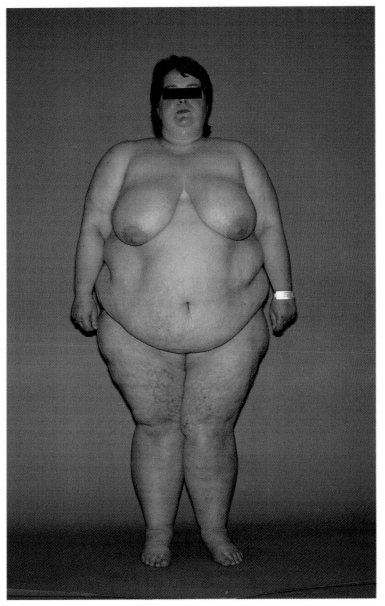

Fig. 235 Simple obesity

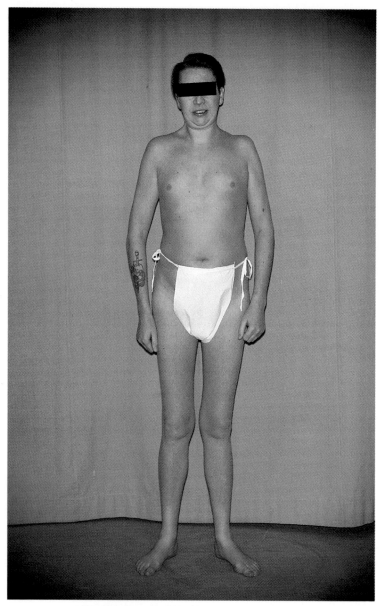

Fig. 236 Eunuchoid habitus: hypopituitarism

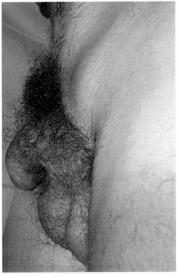

Fig. 237 Inguinal lymphadenopathy

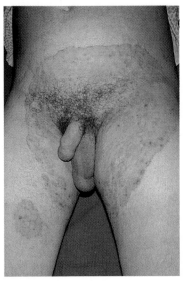

Fig. 238 Tinea cruris

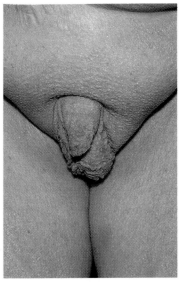

Fig. 239 Hypogonadism

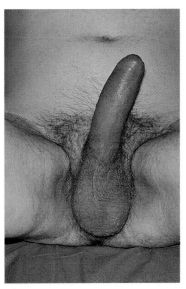

Fig. 240 Priapism

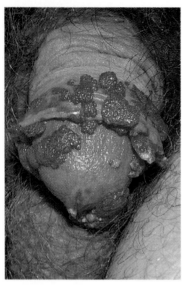

Fig. 241 Penile warts

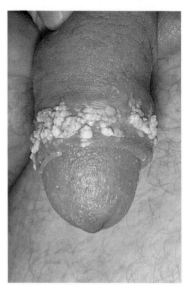

Fig. 242 Penile warts

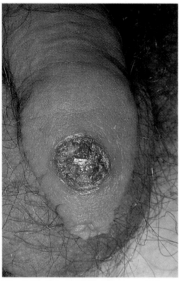

Fig. 243 Primary chancre: syphilis

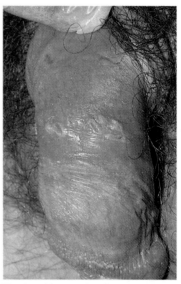

Fig. 244 Herpes simplex

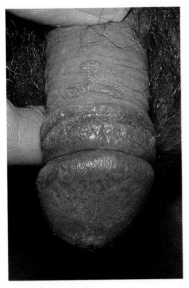

Fig. 245 Psoriasis

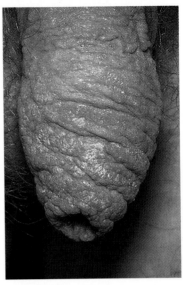

Fig. 246 Lichen planus

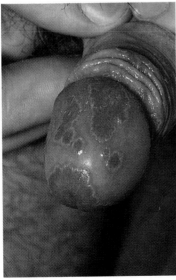

Fig. 247 Circinate balanitis

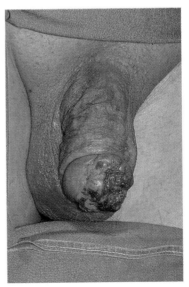

Fig. 248 Carcinoma

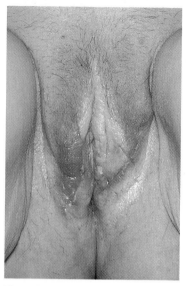

Fig. 249 Lichen sclerosus

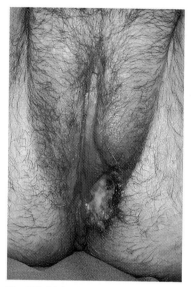

Fig. 250 Vulval ulcer

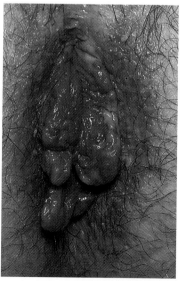

Fig. 251 Prolapsed haemorrhoids

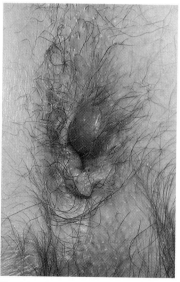

Fig. 252 Thrombosed haemorrhoid

Legs and feet

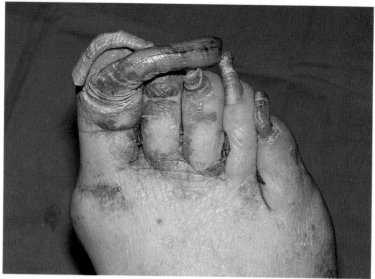

Fig. 253 Onychogryphosis

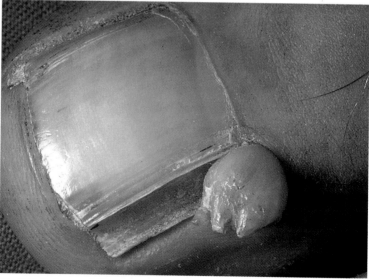

Fig. 254 Subungual fibroma

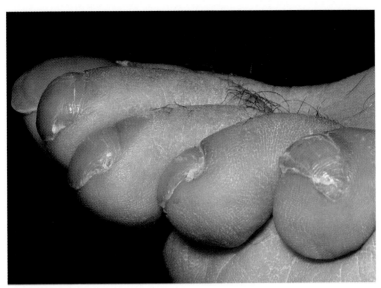

Fig. 255 Clubbing

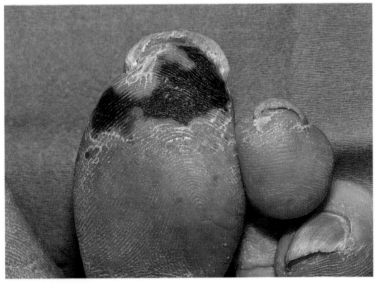

Fig. 256 Vasculitic infarcts

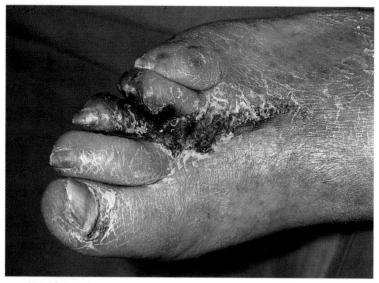

Fig. 257 Digital gangrene

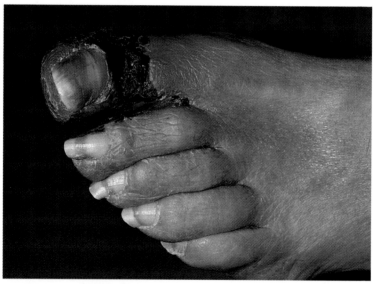

Fig. 258 Digital gangrene

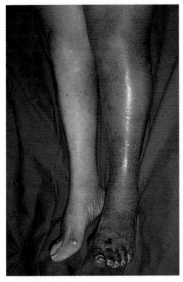

Fig. 259 Arterial gangrene

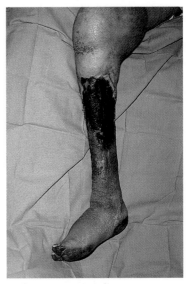

Fig. 260 Arterial gangrene

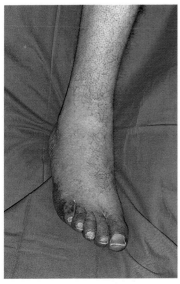

Fig. 261 Venous gangrene

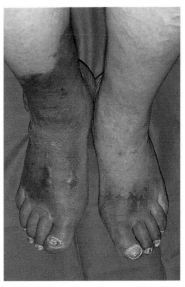

Fig. 262 Venous gangrene

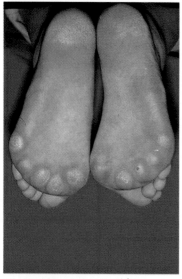

Fig. 263 Rheumatoid arthritis—
metatarsophalangeal subluxations

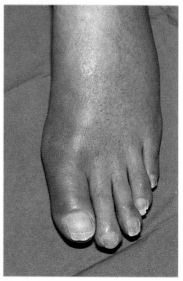

Fig. 264 Acute gout

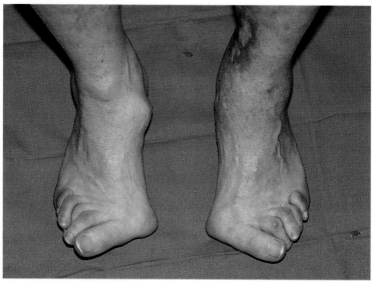

Fig. 265 Hallux valgus

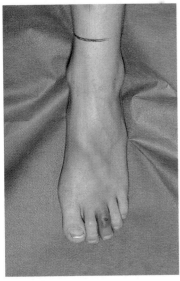

Fig. 266 Lymphangitis

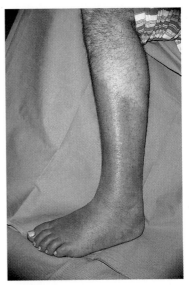

Fig. 267 Cellulitis

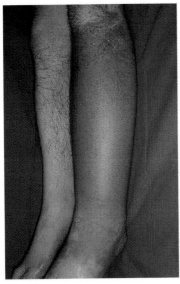

Fig. 268 Cellulitis—acute

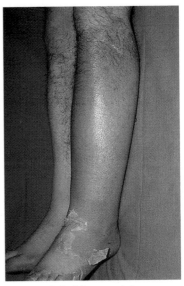

Fig. 269 Cellulitis—resolving

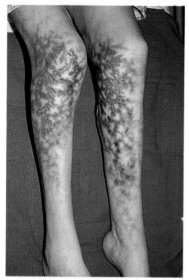

Fig. 270 Erythema ab igne

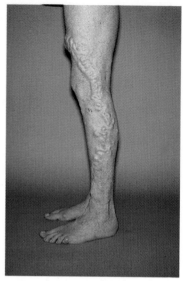

Fig. 271 Varicose veins

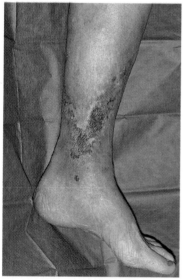

Fig. 272 Varicose ulcer

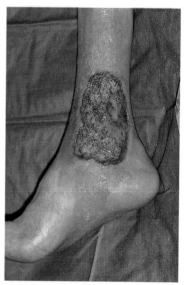

Fig. 273 Varicose ulcer

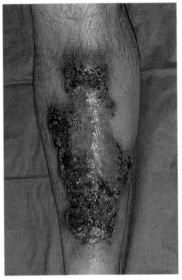

Fig. 274 Vasculitic ulceration

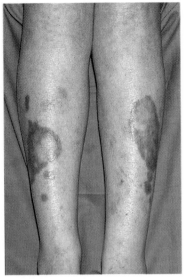

Fig. 275 Necrobiosis lipoidica

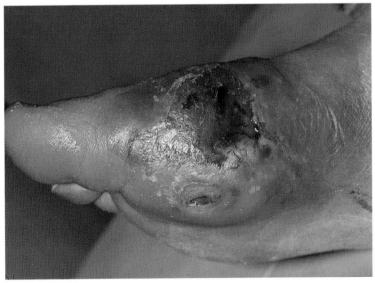

Fig. 276 Trophic ulceration

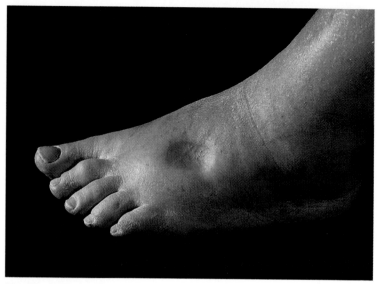

Fig. 277 Pitting oedema

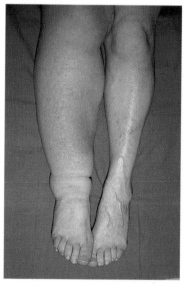

Fig. 278 Lymphoedema

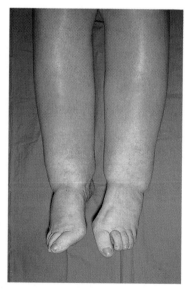

Fig. 279 Lymphoedema

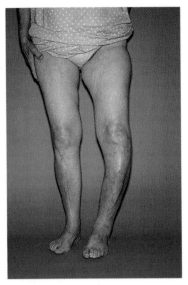

Fig. 280 Paget's disease

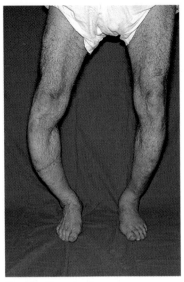

Fig. 281 Paget's disease

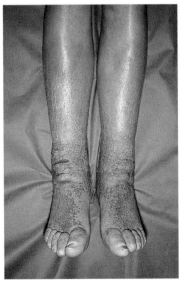

Fig. 282 Pretibial myxoedema

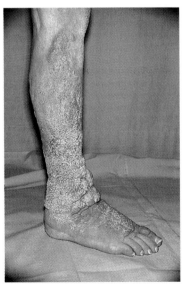

Fig. 283 Pretibial myxoedema

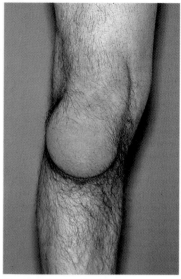

Fig. 284 Prepatellar bursa

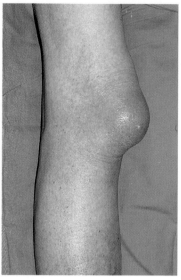

Fig. 285 Prepatellar bursitis

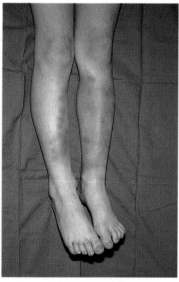

Fig. 286 Erythema nodosum

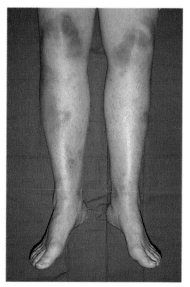

Fig. 287 Erythema nodosum

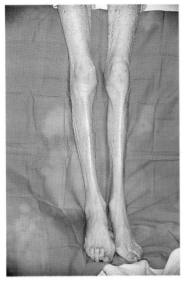

Fig. 288 Muscle wasting—cachexia

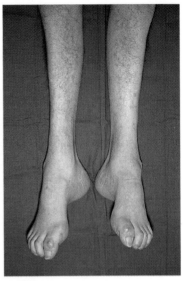

Fig. 289 Muscle wasting—neuropathic

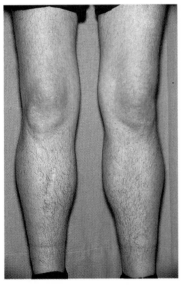

Fig. 290 Muscular dystrophy—pseudohypertrophy

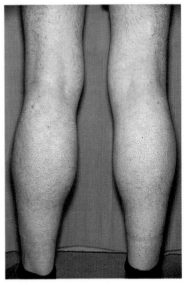

Fig. 291 Muscular dystrophy—pseudohypertrophy

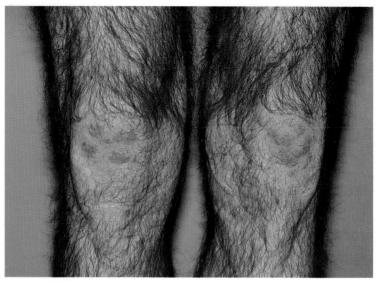

Fig. 292 Xanthomata

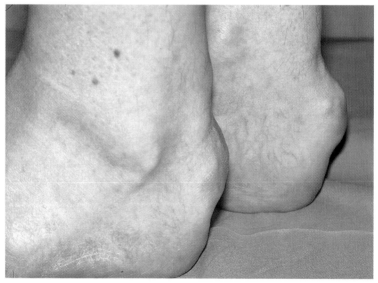

Fig. 293 Xanthomata

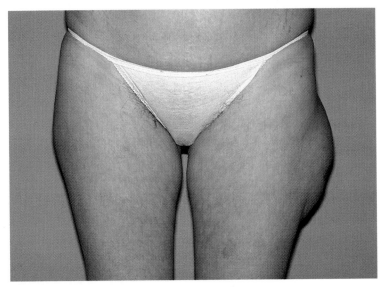

Fig. 294 Lipohypertrophy

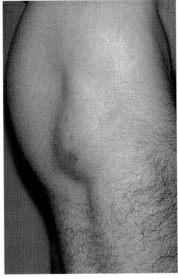

Fig. 295 Lipohypertrophy

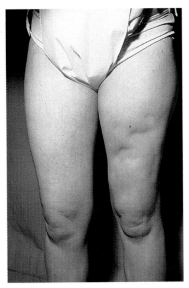

Fig. 296 Lipoatrophy

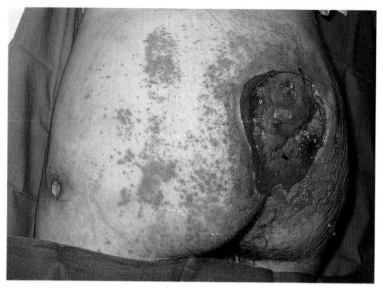

Fig. 297 Decubitus ulcers (pressure sores)

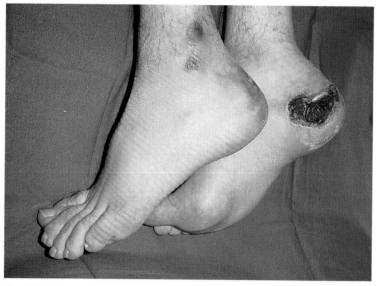

Fig. 298 Decubitus ulcers (pressure sores)

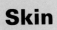

Skin

Fig. 299 Urticarial rash

Fig. 300 Macular rash

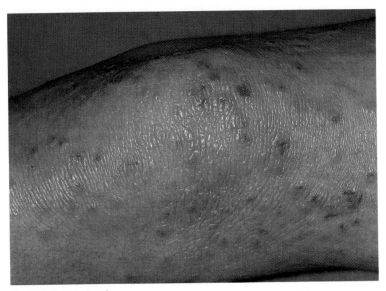

Fig. 301 Papular rash

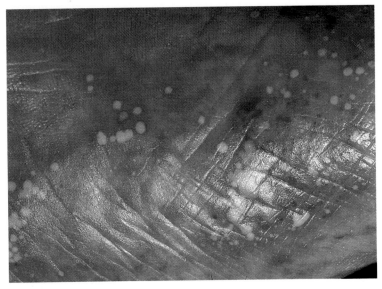

Fig. 302 Pustular rash

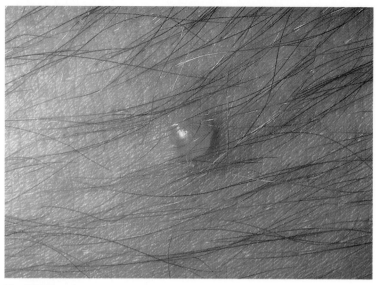

Fig. 303 Vesicle

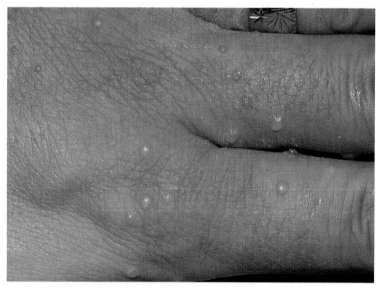

Fig. 304 Vesicles

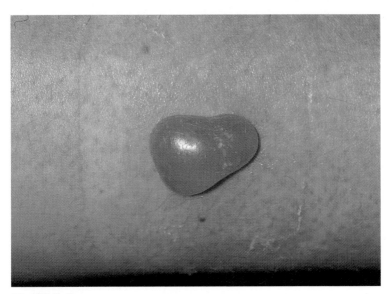

Fig. 305 Bulla

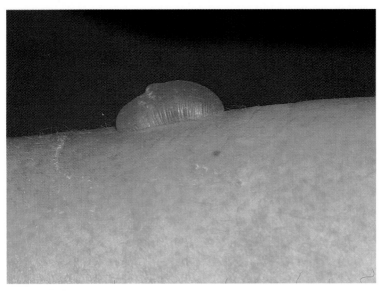

Fig. 306 Bulla

119

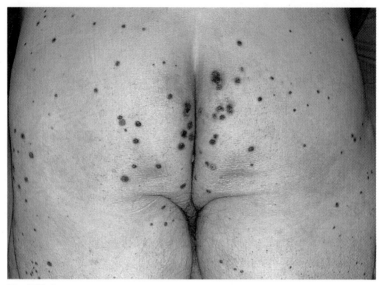

Fig. 307 Purpura—vasculitic

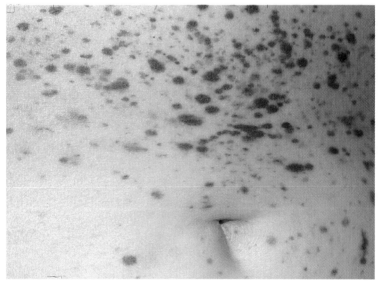

Fig. 308 Purpura—thrombocytopenic

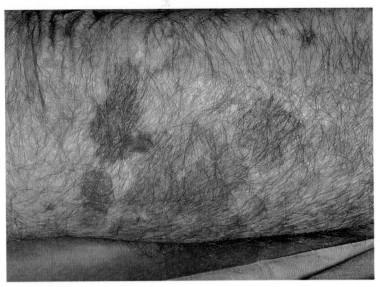

Fig. 309 Purpura—senile

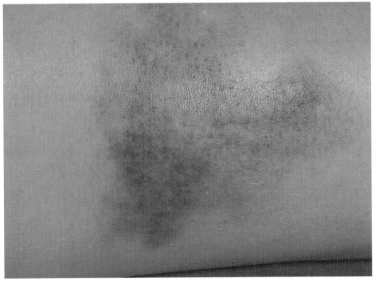

Fig. 310 Bruising

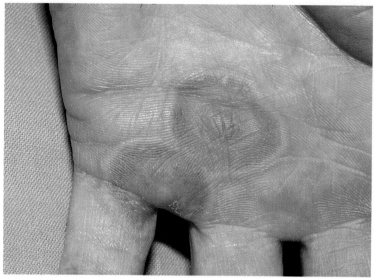

Fig. 311 Target lesions

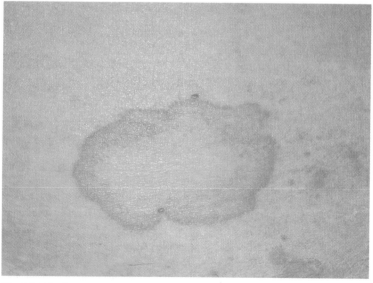

Fig. 312 Erythema marginatum

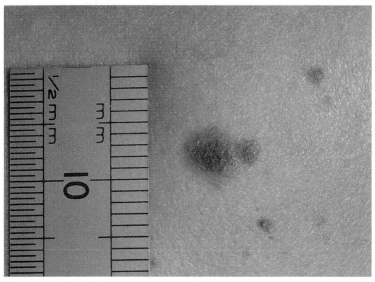

Fig. 313 Pigmented naevi

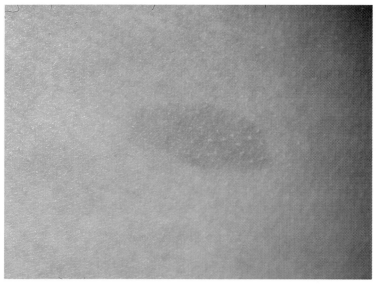

Fig. 314 Café au lait patch

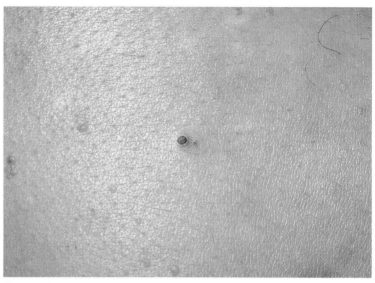

Fig. 315 Comedones

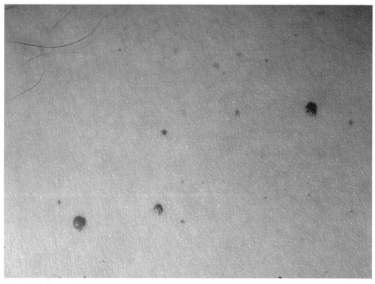

Fig. 316 Campbell de Morgan spots

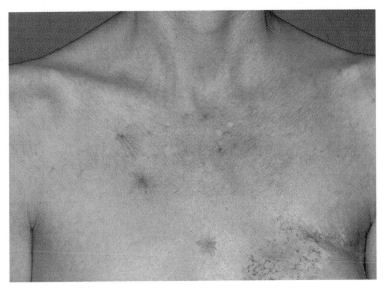

Fig. 317 Spider naevi

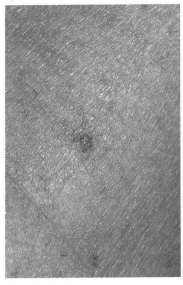

Fig. 318 Spider naevus

Fig. 319 Spider naevus—blanching on pressure

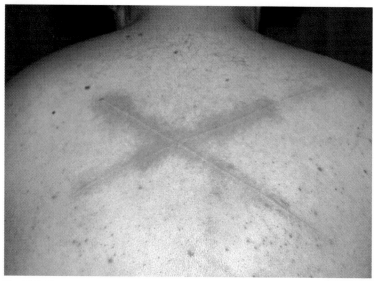

Fig. 320 Dermographism

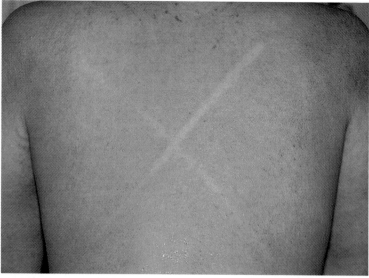

Fig. 321 Dermographism

Fig. 322 Ichthyosis

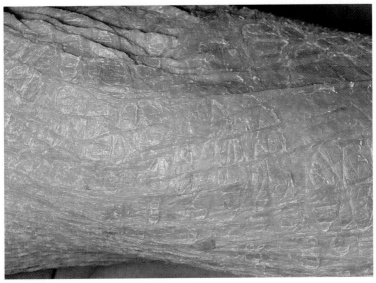

Fig. 323 Ichthyosis

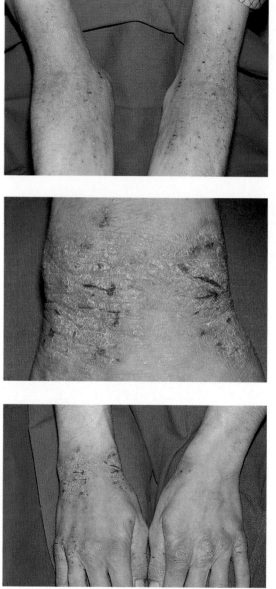

Fig. 324 Atopic eczema

Fig. 325 Atopic eczema

Fig. 326 Atopic eczema

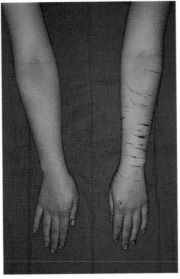

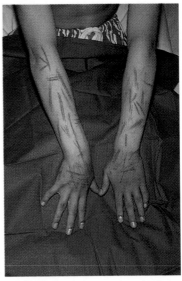

Fig. 327 Dermatitis artefacta (self-mutilation)

Fig. 328 Dermatitis artefacta (self-mutilation)

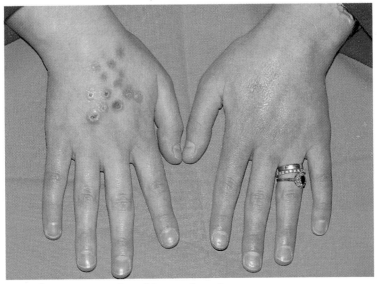

Fig. 329 Dermatitis artefacta (cigarette burns)

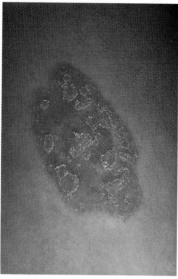

Fig. 330 Psoriasis

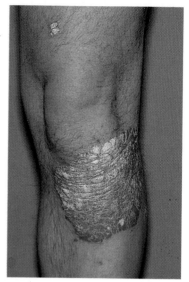

Fig. 331 Psoriasis

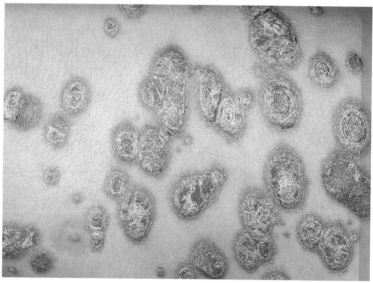

Fig. 332 Psoriasis

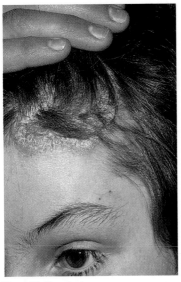

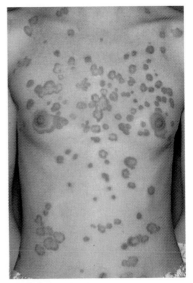

Fig. 333 Psoriasis

Fig. 334 Psoriasis

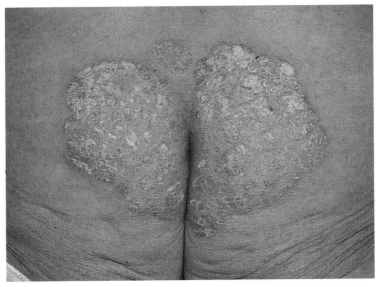

Fig. 335 Psoriasis

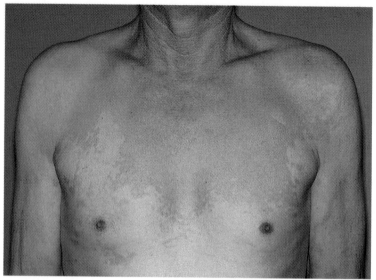

Fig. 336 Pityriasis versicolor

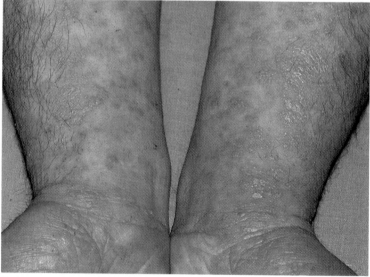

Fig. 337 Lichen planus

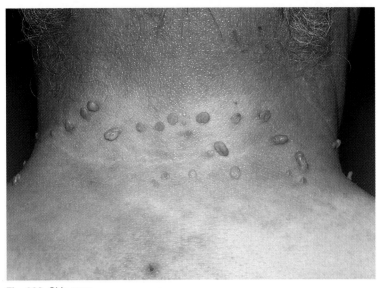

Fig. 338 Skin tags

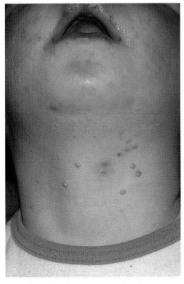

Fig. 339 Molluscum contagiosum

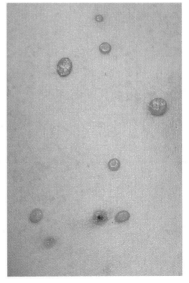

Fig. 340 Molluscum contagiosum

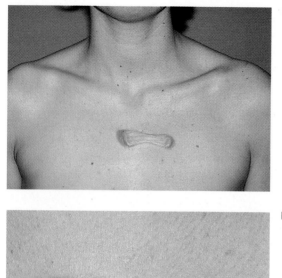

Fig. 341 Keloid scar

Fig. 342 Keloid scar

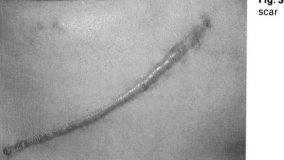

Fig. 343 Hypertrophic scar

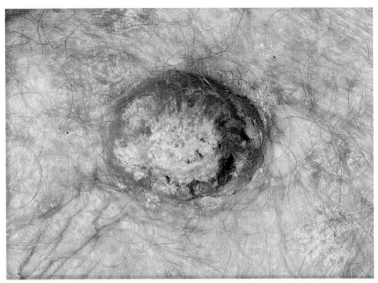

Fig. 344 Keratoacanthoma

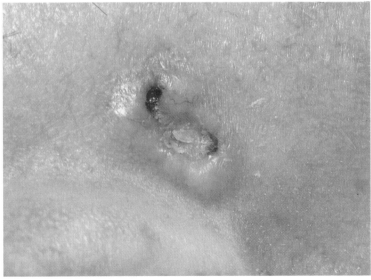

Fig. 345 Basal cell carcinoma (rodent ulcer)

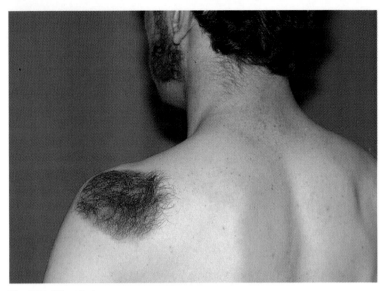

Fig. 346 Giant hairy naevus

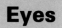

Eyes

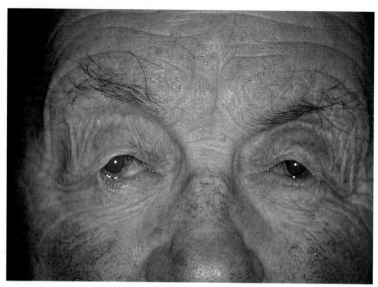

Fig. 347 Cataract—black pupillary reflex

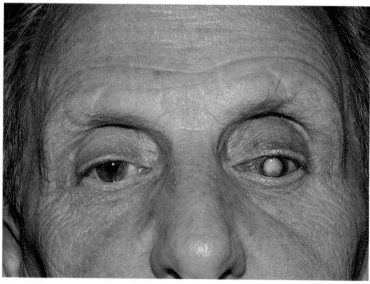

Fig. 348 Cataract—white pupillary reflex

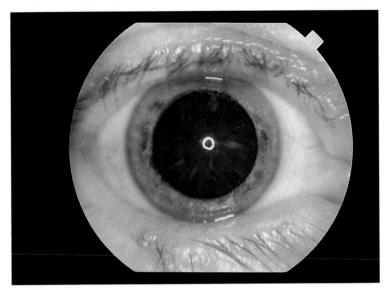

Fig. 349 Cortical cataract

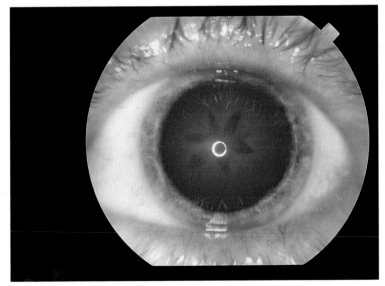

Fig. 350 Stellate cataract

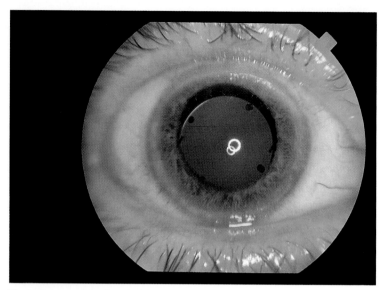

Fig. 351 Intraocular lens implant

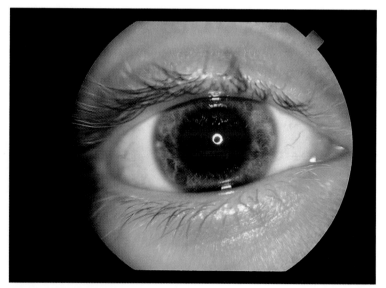

Fig. 352 Dislocated lens

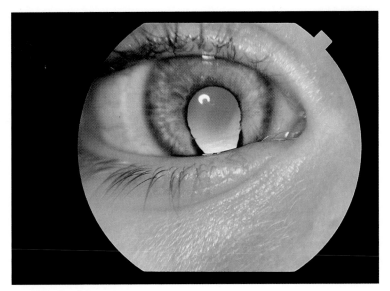

Fig. 353 Coloboma of iris

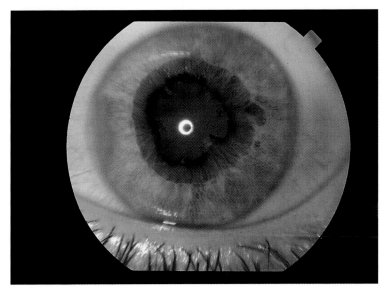

Fig. 354 Irregular pupil: iritis

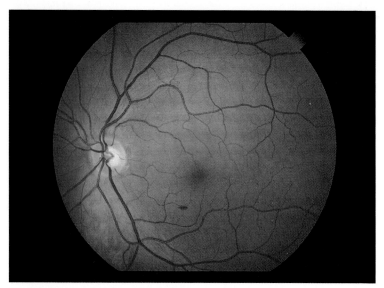

Fig. 355 Nerve-fibre layer (flame) haemorrhage

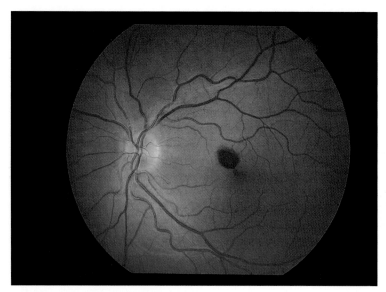

Fig. 356 Intraretinal (blot) haemorrhage

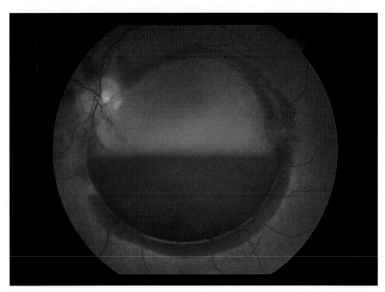

Fig. 357 Preretinal (subhyaloid) haemorrhage

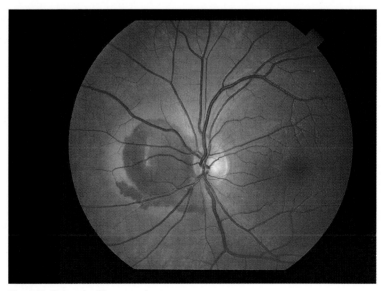

Fig. 358 Subretinal haemorrhage

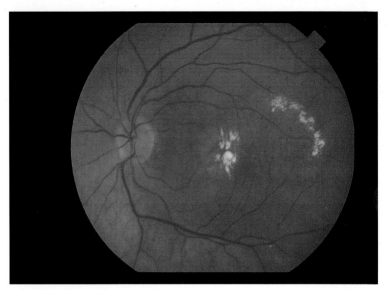

Fig. 359 Hard exudates

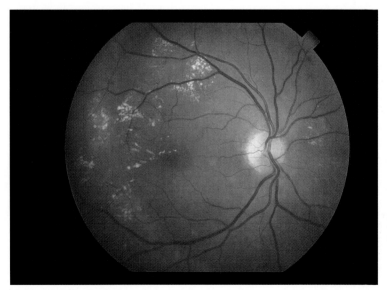

Fig. 360 Hard exudates

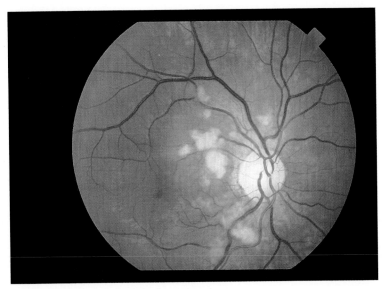

Fig. 361 Cotton wool spots (soft exudates)

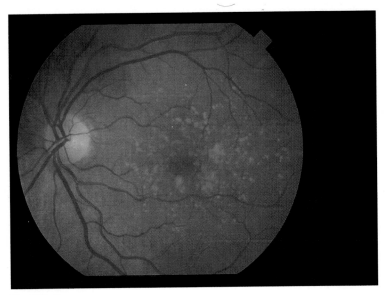

Fig. 362 Drusen

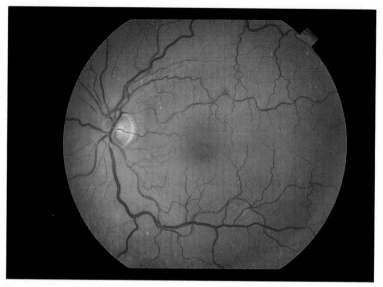

Fig. 363 Hypertensive retinopathy—arteriovenous changes

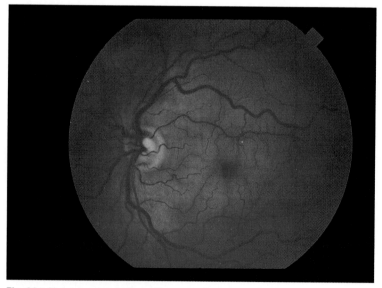

Fig. 364 Hypertensive retinopathy—arteriovenous changes

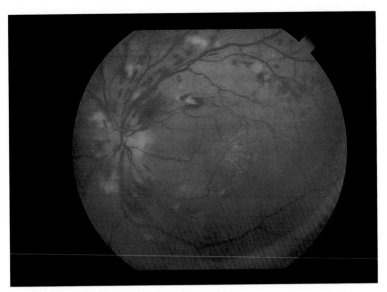

Fig. 365 Hypertensive retinopathy—accelerated hypertension

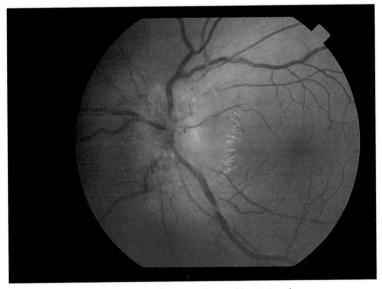

Fig. 366 Hypertensive retinopathy—accelerated hypertension

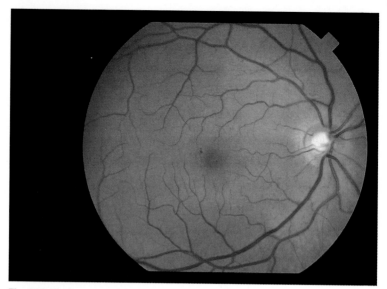

Fig. 367 Background diabetic retinopathy—minimal

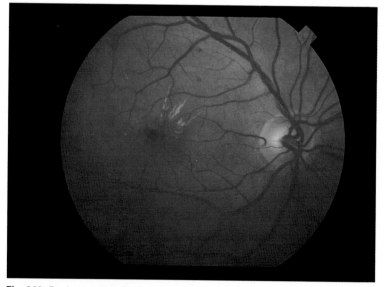

Fig. 368 Background diabetic retinopathy—mild

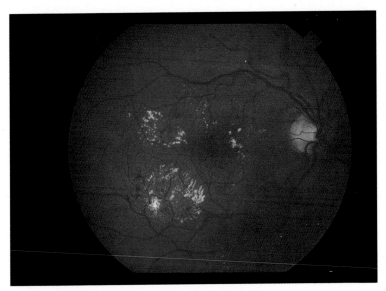

Fig. 369 Background diabetic retinopathy—moderate

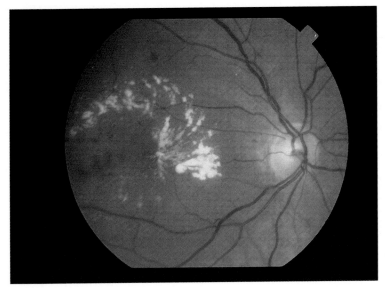

Fig. 370 Diabetic maculopathy

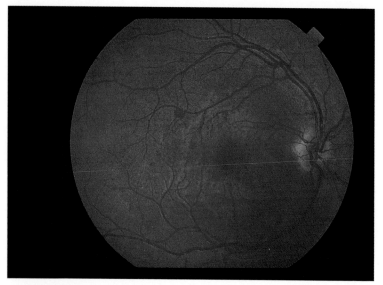

Fig. 371 Background diabetic retinopathy—'dots' and small 'blots'

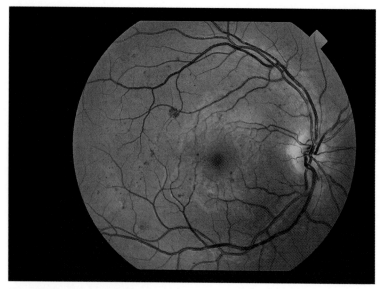

Fig. 372 Background diabetic retinopathy—red-free (green) illumination; compare with Figure 371

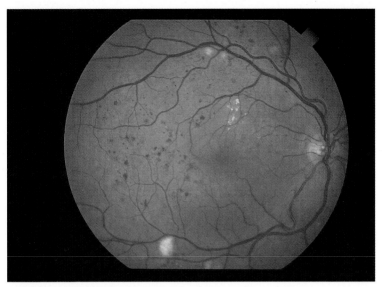

Fig. 373 Preproliferative diabetic retinopathy—cotton wool spots

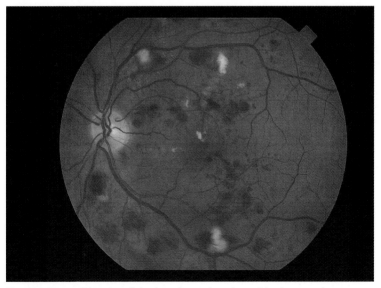

Fig. 374 Preproliferative diabetic retinopathy—large blot haemorrhages

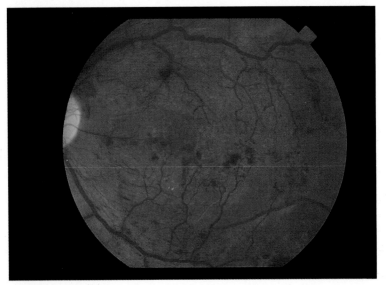

Fig. 375 Preproliferative diabetic retinopathy—beaded major vein

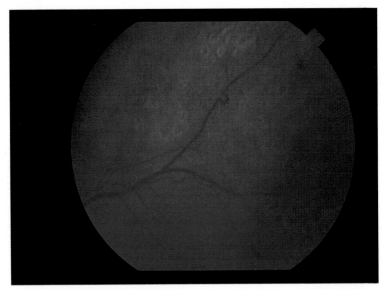

Fig. 376 Preproliferative diabetic retinopathy—venous loop (omega loop)

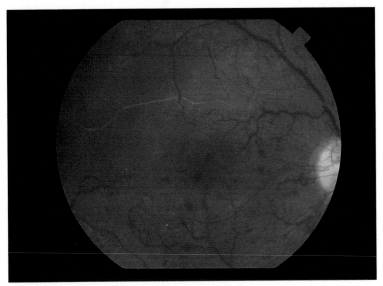

Fig. 377 Preproliferative diabetic retinopathy—ghost vessel

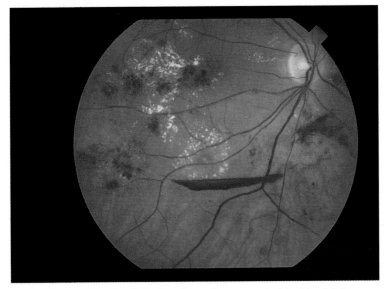

Fig. 378 Preproliferative diabetic retinopathy—preretinal (subhyaloid) haemorrhage

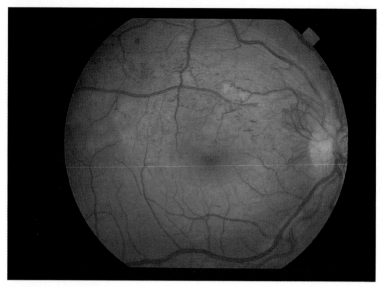

Fig. 379 Proliferative diabetic retinopathy—disc new vessels

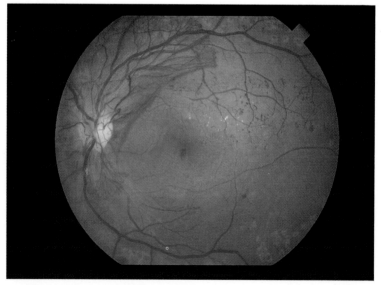

Fig. 380 Proliferative diabetic retinopathy—disc new vessels

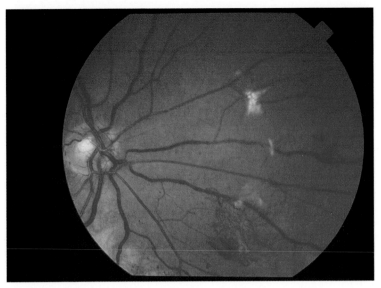

Fig. 381 Proliferative diabetic retinopathy—peripheral new vessels

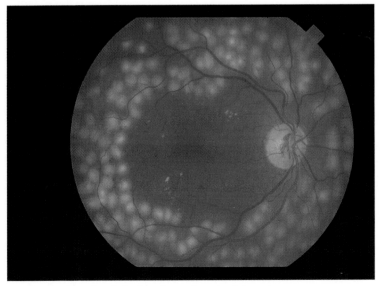

Fig. 382 Proliferative diabetic retinopathy—fresh laser burns

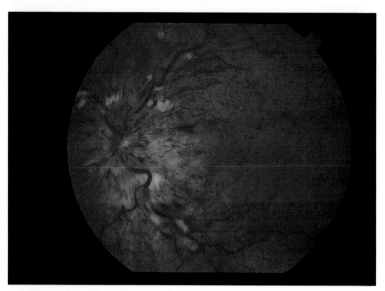

Fig. 383 Central retinal vein occlusion

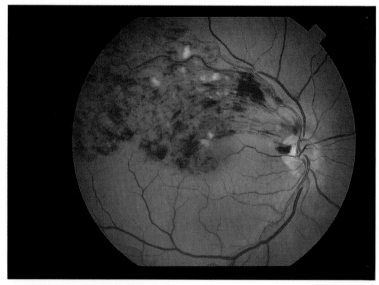

Fig. 384 Branch retinal vein occlusion

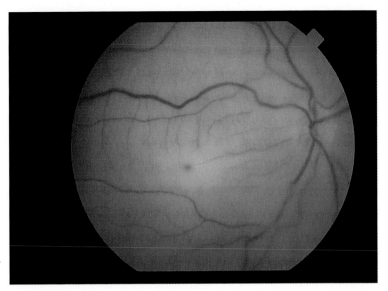

Fig. 385 Central retinal artery occlusion

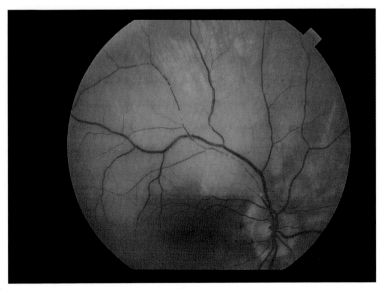

Fig. 386 Branch retinal artery occlusion

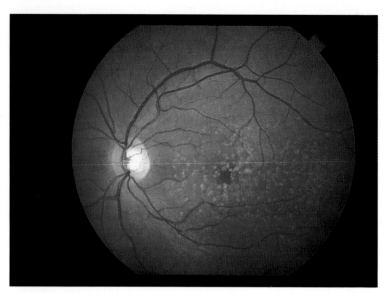

Fig. 387 Senile macular degeneration—drusen

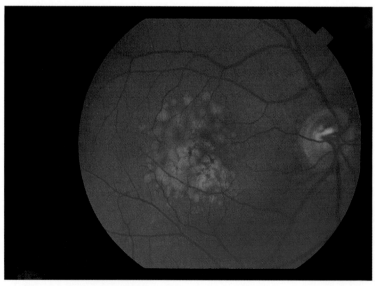

Fig. 388 Senile macular degeneration—atrophic ('dry')

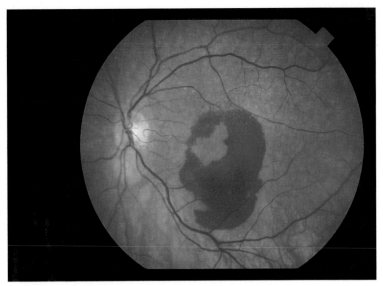

Fig. 389 Senile macular degeneration—disciform ('wet')

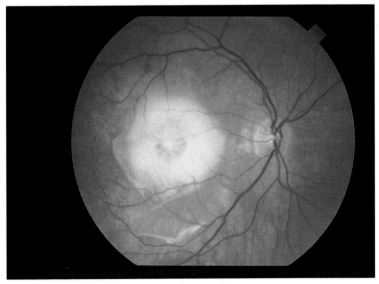

Fig. 390 Senile macular degeneration—disciform scar

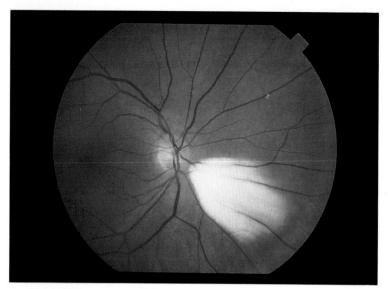

Fig. 391 Myelinated nerve fibres

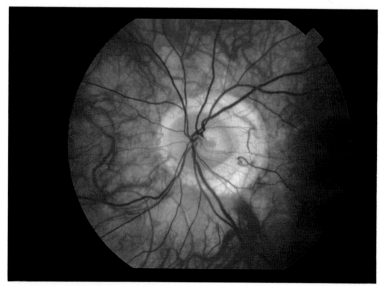

Fig. 392 Myopic disc

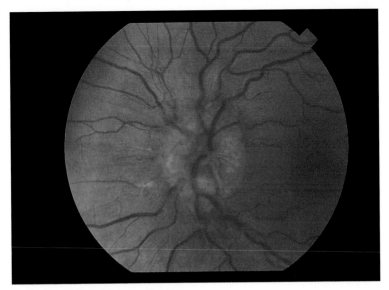

Fig. 393 Swollen disc—papilloedema

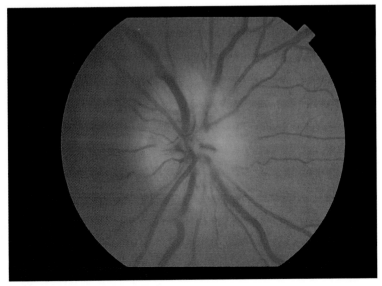

Fig. 394 Swollen disc—papillitis

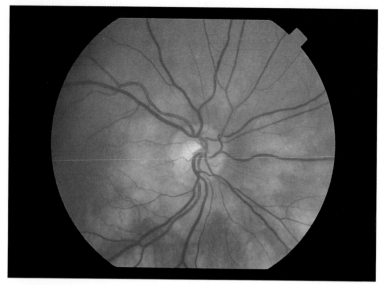

Fig. 395 Normal optic disc cup

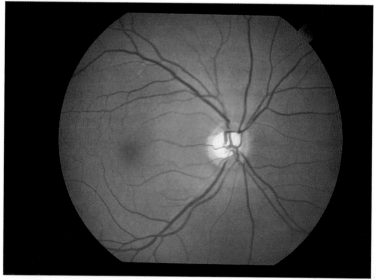

Fig. 396 Suspicious disc cupping

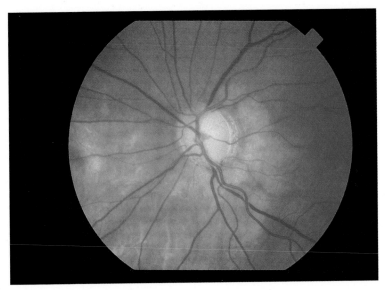

Fig. 397 Pathological disc cupping

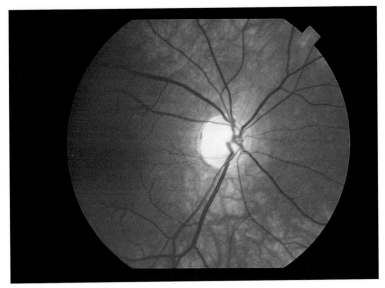

Fig. 398 Optic atrophy

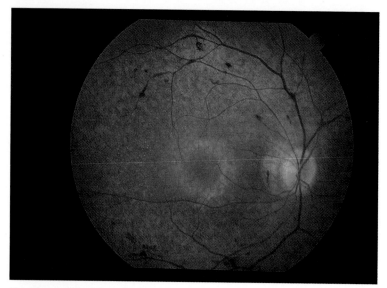

Fig. 399 Retinitis pigmentosa

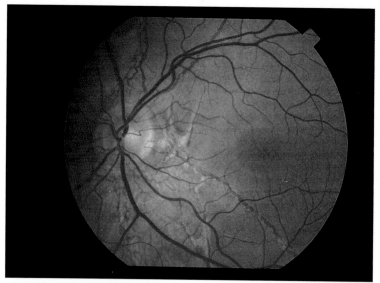

Fig. 400 Angioid streaks

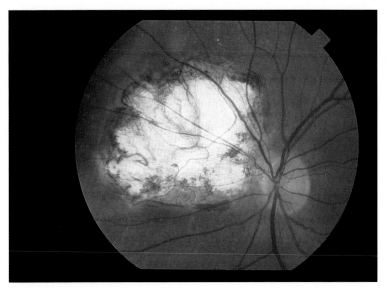

Fig. 401 Toxoplasma choroiditis

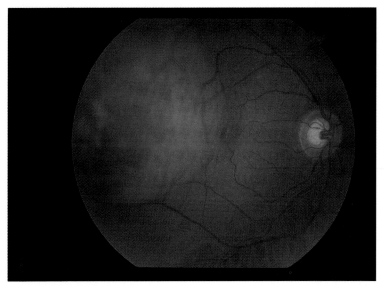

Fig. 402 Choroidal tumour

International glossary

- Pour que ce livre soit plus accessible à un marché international, on a traduit chacune des légendes en français

- Um dieses Buch einem internationalen Markt zugänglich zu machen, ist jede Unterschrift ins Deutsch übersetzt worden

- Para posibilitar que este libro sea utilidado en un mercado internacional, cada una de las legendas ha sido tradvirda al español

Head and neck

Fig. 1 Left facial palsy—lower motor neurone

- Paralysie faciale côté gauche—
  neurone motrice inférieure

- Linksseitige Gesichtslähmung—
  unteres Motorneuron

- Parálisis facial lado izquierdo—
  neurona motriz inferior

Fig. 2 Left facial palsy—closing eyes

- Paralysie faciale côté gauche—
  fermant les yeux

- Linksseitige Gesichtslähmung—
  Lidschluß

- Parálisis facial lado izquierdo—
  cerrando los ojos

Fig. 3 Left facial palsy—upper motor neurone

- Paralysie faciale côté gauche—
  neurone motrice supérieure

- Linksseitige Gesichtslähmung—
  oberes Motorneuron

- Parálisis facial lado izquierdo—
  neurona motriz superior

Fig. 4 Left facial palsy—closing eyes

- Paralysie faciale côté gauche—
  fermant les yeux

- Linksseitige Gesichtslähmung—
  Lidschluß

- Parálisis facial lado izquierdo—
  cerrando los ojos

Fig. 5 Jaundice

- Ictére

- Ikterus

- Ictericia

Fig. 6 Jaundice

- Ictére

- Ikterus

- Ictericia

Fig. 7 Jaundice

- Ictére

- Ikterus

- Ictericia

Fig. 8 Telangiectasia

- Télangiectasie

- Teleangiektasie

- Telangiectasia

Fig. 9 Butterfly rash

- Éruption en papillon
- Schmetterlingsförmiger Rash
- Erupción en forma de mariposa

Fig. 10 Butterfly rash

- Éruption en papillon
- Schmetterlingsförmiger Rash
- Erupción en forma de mariposa

Fig. 11 Pallor

- Pâleur
- Pallor (Blässe)
- Palidez

Fig. 12 Vitiligo

- Leucodermie
- Vitiligo
- Vitíligo

Fig. 13 Malar flush

- Rougeur de la pommette
- Wangenflush
- Enrojecimiento de las mejillas

Fig. 14 Photosensitive rash

- Éruption photosensible
- Rash nach Photosensibilisierung
- Erupción fotosensible

Fig. 15 Acne vulgaris

- Acné vulgaire
- Acne vulgaris
- Acne vulgar

Fig. 16 Acne vulgaris

- Acné vulgaire
- Acne vulgaris
- Acne vulgar

Fig. 17 Acne scarring

- Cicatrices de l'acné
- Acne mit Narbenbildung
- Cicatrices producidas por el acne

Fig. 18 Rosacea

- Rosacée
- Rosacea
- Rosácea

Fig. 19 Rosacea

- Rosacée
- Rosacea
- Rosácea

Fig. 20 Rhinophyma

- Rhinophyma
- Rhinophym
- Rinofima

Fig. 21 Chickenpox

- Varicelle
- Varicellen
- Varicela

Fig. 22 Kaposi's varicelliform eruption

- Éruption varicelliforme de Kaposi
- Kaposi Dermatitis
- Enfermedad de Kaposi

Fig. 23 Adenoma sebaceum

- Adénome sébacé
- Adenoma sebaceum
- Adenoma sebáceo

Fig. 24 Ophthalmic herpes zoster

- Zona ophtalmique
- Herpes zoster des Auges
- Herpes zóster oftálmico

Fig. 25 Maxillary herpes zoster

- Zona maxillaire
- Herpes zoster der Maxilla
- Herpes zóster maxilar

Fig. 26 Mandibular herpes zoster

- Zona mandibulaire
- Herpes zoster der Mandibula
- Herpes zóster mandibular

Fig. 27 Post-herpetic scarring

- Cicatrisation post-herpétique
- Narbenbildung nach Herpes
- Cicatrización post-herpética

Fig. 28 Facial cellulitis

- Cellulite faciale
- Zellulitis des Gesichts
- Celulitis facial

Fig. 29 Facial swelling

- Enflure faciale
- Gesichtsschwellung
- Tumefacción facial

Fig. 30 Parotid swelling

- Inflammation du parotide
- Parotisschwellung
- Inflamación de la glándula parótida

Fig. 31 Branchial cyst

- Kyste branchiale
- Branchiogene Zyste
- Quiste branquial

Fig. 32 Pagetic skull

- Maladie osseuse de Paget-crâne
- Schädel bei M. Paget
- Enfermedad de Paget-cráneo

Fig. 33 Cavernous haemangioma (port-wine stain)

- Hémangiome caverneuse (tache de vin)
- Hämangioma cavernosum (Portweinfleck)
- Hemangioma cavernoso (mancha de vino)

Fig. 34 Micrognathia

- Micrognathie
- Micrognathie
- Micrognatia

Fig. 35 Prognathia

- Prognathiome
- Prognathie
- Prognatismo

Fig. 36 Thyrotoxicosis

- Thyrotoxicose
- Thyrotoxicose
- Tirotoxicosis

Fig. 37 Goitre

- Goitre
- Struma
- Bocio

Fig. 38 Goitre

- Goitre
- Struma
- Bocio

Fig. 39 Thyroglossal cyst

- Kyste thyréoglosse

- Thyreoglossus-Zyste

- Quiste tiroglingual

Fig. 40 Hypothyroidism

- Hypothyroïdie

- Hypothyreose

- Hipotiroidismo

Fig. 41 Hypothyroidism

- Hypothyroïdie

- Hypothyreose

- Hipotiroidismo

Fig. 42 Hypothyroidism—untreated

- Hypothyroïdie—sans traitement

- Hypothyreodismus—vor
  Behandlung

- Hipotiroidismo—sin tratamiento

Fig. 43 Hypothyroidism—treated

- Hypothyroïdie—avec traitement

- Hypothyreodismus nach
  Behandlung

- Hipotiroidismo—con tratamiento

Fig. 44 Hirsutism

- Hirsutie

- Hirsutismus

- Hirsutismo

Fig. 45 Hirsutism

- Hirsutie

- Hirsutismus

- Hirsutismo

Fig. 46 Hirsutism

- Hirsutie

- Hirsutismus

- Hirsutismo

**Fig. 47 Cushing's syndrome—
spontaneous**

- Syndrome de Cushing—spontané

- Cushing-Syndrom—spontan

- Síndrome de Cushing—
  espontáneo

**Fig. 48 Cushing's syndrome—
iatrogenous**

- Syndrome de Cushing—
  iatrogénique

- Cushing-Syndrom—iatrogen

- Síndrome de Cushing—iatrógeno

Fig. 49 Addisonian pigmentation

- Pigmentation typique de la maladie d'Addison

- Hyperpigmentation bei M. Addison

- Pigmentación caracteristic de la enfermedad de Addison

Fig. 50 Hypopituitarism

- Hypopituitarisme

- Hypopituitarismus

- Hipopituitarismo

Fig. 51 Acromegaly

- Acromégalie

- Akromegalie

- Acromegalía

Fig. 52 Acromegaly

- Acromégalie

- Akromegalie

- Acromegalía

Fig. 53 Acromegaly

- Acromégalie

- Akromegalie

- Acromegalía

Fig. 54 Progressive systemic sclerosis

- Sclérose systémique progréssive

- Progressive Systemsclerose

- Esclerosis sistémica progresiva

Fig. 55 Myotonic dystrophy

- Dystrophie myotonique

- Myotonia dystrophica

- Distrofía miotónica

Fig. 56 Neck webbing

- Con palmé

- Halsband

- Cvello palmeado

Fig. 57 Left sixth-nerve palsy—looking left

- Paralysie du sixième nerf gauche—regardant à gauche

- Linksseitige Abducenslähmung—Blick nach links

- Parálisis del nervio sexto izquierdo—mirando hacia la izquierda

Fig. 58 Left sixth-nerve palsy—looking ahead

- Paralysie du sixième nerf gauche—regardant tout droit

- Linksseitige Abducenslähmung—Blick nach vorn

- Parálisis del nervio sexto izquierdo—mirando hacia delante

Fig. 59 Left sixth-nerve palsy—looking right

- Paralysie du sixième nerf gauche—regardant à droite

- Linksseitige Abducenslähmung—Blick nach rechts

- Parálisis del nervio sexto izquierdo—mirando hacia la derecha

Fig. 60 Left third-nerve palsy—complete ptosis

- Paralysie du troisième nerf gauche—ptosis totale

- Linksseitige Oculomotoriuslähmung—komplette Ptosis

- Parálisis del nervio tercero izquierdo—ptosis total

Fig. 61 Left third-nerve palsy—looking right

- Paralysie du troisième nerf gauche—regardant à droite

- Linksseitige Oculomotoriuslähmung—Blick nach rechts

- Parálisis del nervio tercero izquierdo—mirando hacia la derecha

Fig. 62 Left third-nerve palsy—pupillary dilatation

- Paralysie du troisième nerf gauche—dilatation pupillaire

- Linksseitige Oculomotoriuslähmung—Pupillenerweiterung

- Parálisis del nervio tercero izquierdo—dilatación de la pupila

Fig. 63 Xanthelasmata

- Xanthélasmes

- Xanthelasmen

- Xanthelasmas

Fig. 64 Xanthelasmata

- Xanthélasmes

- Xanthelasmen

- Xanthelasmas

Fig. 65 Xanthelasmata and corneal arcus

- Xanthélasmes et arcade cornéenne

- Xanthelasmen und Korneabogen

- Xanthelasmas y arco corneal

Fig. 66 Xanthelasmata

- Xanthélasmes

- Xanthelasmen

- Xanthelasmas

Fig. 67 Xanthelasmata

- Xanthélasmes

- Xanthelasmen

- Xanthelasmas

Fig. 68 Dysthyroid eye disease: upper and lower lid retraction

- Maladie dysthyroïdique des yeux: rétraction des paupiéres supérieure et inférieure

- Augenbeteiligung bei Dysthyreose: Retraktion von Ober und Unterlid

- Distiroidismo ocular: retracción del párpado superior e inferior

Fig. 69 Dysthyroid eye disease: proptosis

- Maladie dysthyroïdique des yeux: prolapsus

- Augenbeteiligung bei Dysthyreose: Proptosis

- Distiroidismo ocular: proptosis

Fig. 70 Bilateral ectropion

- Ectropion bilatéral

- Bilaterales Ektropium

- Ectropión bilateral

Fig. 71 Entropion

- Entropion

- Entropium

- Entropión

Fig. 72 Ptosis—congenital

- Ptosis—congénitale

- Ptosis—kongenital

- Ptosis—congénita

Fig. 73 Ptosis—acquired: Horner's syndrome

- Ptosis—acquise: syndrome de Bernard-Horner

- Ptosis—erworben: Horner-Syndrom

- Ptosis—adquirida: síndrome de Horner

Fig. 74 Myasthenia gravis—bilateral ptosis

- Myasthénie grave—ptosis bilatérale

- Myasthenia gravis—beidseitige Ptosis

- Miastemia grave—ptosis bilateral

Fig. 75 Myasthenia gravis—after anticholinesterase injection

- Myasthénie grave—après injection d'anticholinestérase

- Myasthenia gravis—nach Anticholinesteraseinjektion

- Miastemia grave—tras inyección de anticolinesterasa

Fig. 76 Dacryocystitis

- Dacriocystite

- Dacrozystitis

- Dacriocistitis

Fig. 77 Orbital cellulitis

- Cellulite orbitaire

- Orbitale Zellulitis

- Celulitis orbital

Fig. 78 Subconjunctival haemorrhage—spontaneous

- Hémorragie subconjonctivale— spontanée

- Subconjunktivale Blutung— spontan

- Hemorragia subconjuntival— espontánea

Fig. 79 Subconjunctival haemorrhage—traumatic

- Hémorragie subconjonctivale— traumatique

- Subconjunktivale Blutung— traumatisch

- Hemorragia subconjuntival— traumática

Fig. 80 Conjunctivitis—limbal pallor

- Conjonctivite—pâleur du limbe

- Konjunktivitis—blaßer Limbus

- Conjuntivitis—palides del limbo

Fig. 81 Iritis—limbal injection

- Iritis—injection limbale

- Iritis—Gefäßinjektion des Limbus

- Iritis—inyección limbal

Fig. 82 Episcleritis

- Épisclérite

- Episkleritis

- Episcleritis

Fig. 83 Scleritis—nodular

- Sclérite—nodulaire
- Skleritis—nodulär
- Esclerotitis—nodular

Fig. 84 Scleritis—diffuse

- Sclérite—répandue
- Skleritis—diffus
- Esclerotitis—difusa

Fig. 85 Pterygium

- Ptérigion
- Pterygium
- Pterigion

Fig. 86 Pinguecula

- Pinguécula
- Pinguecula
- Pinguécula

Fig. 87 Scleromalacia

- Scléromalacie
- Skleromalacie
- Escleromalacia

Fig. 88 Hyphaema

- Hypéma
- Hyphäma
- Hipema

Fig. 89 Hypopyon

- Hypopyon
- Hypopyon
- Hipópion

Fig. 90 Basal cell carcinoma (rodent ulcer)

- Épithélioma basocellulaire (ulcus rodens)
- Basalzellkarzinom (Ulcus rodens)
- Carcinoma basocelular (ulcus rodens)

Fig. 91 Malignant melanoma

- Mélanome malin
- Malignes Melanom
- Melanosis lenticular

Fig. 92 Lentigo maligna

- Mélanose lenticulaire progressive de Pick
- Lentigo maligna
- Peca maligna

Fig. 93 Herpes simplex labialis

- Herpés labial
- Herpes simplex labialis
- Herpes simple labial

Fig. 94 Herpes simplex labialis

- Herpés labial
- Herpes simplex labialis
- Herpes simple labial

Fig. 95 Angular stomatitis

- Perléche
- Stomatitis angularis (Perléche)
- Estomatitis angular

Fig. 96 Angular stomatitis

- Perléche
- Stomatitis angularis (Perléche)
- Estomatitis angular

Fig. 97 Central cyanosis

- Cyanose centrale
- Zentrale Zyanose
- Cianosis central

Fig. 98 Central cyanosis

- Cyanose centrale
- Zentrale Zyanose
- Cianosis central

Fig. 99 Buccal ulceration

- Ulcération buccale
- Wangenulzeration
- Ulceración bucal

Fig. 100 Leukoplakia

- Leucoplasie
- Leukoplakie
- Leucoplaquia

Fig. 101 Pigmented spots: Peutz-Jehger's syndrome

- Taches pigmentées: lentigino-polypose digestive
- Pigmentflecken: Peutz-Jehgers Syndrom
- Manchas pigmentadas: síndrome de Peutz

Fig. 102 Dental caries

- Carie dentaire
- Zahnkaries
- Caries dental

Fig. 103 Tetracycline staining

- Taches de tétracycline
- Verfärbung bei Tetrazyclingabe
- Manchas de tetraciclina

Fig. 104 Gum hyperplasia

- Hyperplasie des gencives
- Zahnfleischhyperplasie
- Hiperplasia de las encías

Fig. 105 Candidiasis

- Candidiase
- Candidiasis
- Oidiomicosis

Fig. 106 Hereditary haemorrhagic telangiectasia

- Maladie de Rendu-Osler
- Hereditäre hämorrhagische Teleangiektasie
- Enfermedad de Rendu-Osler-Weber

Fig. 107 Pallor

- Pâleur
- Pallor (Blässe)
- Palidez

Fig. 108 Geographic tongue

- Langue géographique
- Landkartenzunge (Exfoliatio areata linguae)
- Lengua geográfica

Fig. 109 Atrophic glossitis

- Glossite atrophique
- Atrophische Glossitis
- Glositis atrófica

Fig. 110 Left twelfth-nerve palsy

- Paralysie du douzième nerf gauche
- Linksseitige Hypoglossuslähmung
- Parálisis del nervio duodécimo izquierdo

Fig. 111 Buccal pigmentation

- Pigmentation buccale
- Wangenpigmentation
- Pigmentación bucal

Fig. 112 Lichen planus

- Lichen planus
- Lichen planus
- Liquen planus

Fig. 113 Candidiasis

- Candidiase
- Candidiasis
- Oidiomicosis

Fig. 114 Herpes zoster

- Zona
- Herpes zoster
- Herpes zóster

Fig. 115 Palatal petechiae

- Pétéchie palatale
- Palatinale Petechien
- Petequia del paladar

Fig. 116 Palatal petechiae

- Pétéchie palatale
- Palatinale Petechien
- Petequia del paladar

Fig. 117 Tonsillitis

- Amygdalite
- Tonsillitis
- Amigdalitis

Fig. 118 Tonsillitis

- Amygdalite
- Tonsillitis
- Amigdalitis

Fig. 119 Alopecia—diffuse

- Calvitie—répandue
- Alopecia—maligna totalis
- Calvicie—difusa

Fig. 120 Alopecia—patchy

- Calvitie—en plaques
- Alopecia areata
- Calvicie—desigual

Fig. 121 Solar keratoses

- Kératoses solaires
- Keratosis solaris
- Queratosis solares

Fig. 122 Sebaceous cyst (wen)

- Kyste sébacé (loupe)
- Seborrhoische Zyste (Grützbeutel)
- Quiste sebáceo (lupia)

Fig. 123 Peripheral cyanosis

- Cyanose périphérique
- Periphere Zyanose
- Cianosis periférica

Fig. 124 Gouty tophi

- Tophus de la goutte
- Gichttophi
- Tofos en la gota

Fig. 125 Contact dermatitis

- Dermatite de contacte
- Kontaktdermatitis
- Dermatitis de contacto

Fig. 126 Contact dermatitis

- Dermatite de contacte
- Kontaktdermatitis
- Dermatitis de contacto

Fig. 127 Distended neck veins

- Distension des veines du cou
- Gestaute Halsvenen
- Venas del cuello dilatadas

Fig. 128 Scrofula

- Écrouelles
- Skrofula (Lymphknoten Tbc)
- Escrófula

Fig. 129 Tracheostomy

- Trachéotomie
- Tracheotomie
- Traqueotomía

Fig. 130 Carbuncle

- Furoncle
- Karbunkel
- Carbunclo

Fig. 131 Nail pitting

- Ongles godées
- Tüpfelnägel
- Huellas de presión en las uñas

Fig. 132 Nail fold infarcts

- Calcification du périonyx
- Nagelwallinfarkte
- Infartos calcáreos en el eponiquio

Fig. 133 Splinter haemorrhages

- Hémorragies causées par des échardes
- Splinterblutung
- Hemorragias producidas por astillas

Fig. 134 Beau's lines

- Sillons unquéaux de Beau
- Beau-Reil Furchen
- Líneas de Beau

Fig. 135 Koilonychia

- Koïlonychie
- Koilonychie
- Coiloniquia

Fig. 136 Clubbing—increased longitudinal curvature

- Doigts hippocratiques—courbure longitudinale exagéré
- Trommelschlegelbildung— verstärkte Längskrümmung
- Dedos hipocrátios—curvatura longitudinal exagerada

Fig. 137 Clubbing—loss of nailbed angle

- Doigts hippocratiques—perte de l'angle du lit de l'ongle
- Trommelschlegelbildung—Verlust des Nagelbettwinkels
- Dedos hipocráticos—périda del ángulo del lecho de la una

Fig. 138 Clubbing—drumstick appearance

- Doigts hippocratiques—en forme de baguette de tambour
- Trommelschlegelfinger
- Dedos hipocráticos—forma de palillos de tambor

Fig. 139 Periungual erythema

- Érythéme periunguéal
- Periunguales Erythem
- Eritema periungueal

Fig. 140 Tar (nicotine) staining

- Taches de nicotine
- Nikotinverfärbung
- Manchas de nicotina

Fig. 141 Nail dystrophy

- Dystrophie unguéale
- Nageldystrophie
- Distrofia ungular

Fig. 142 Onycholysis

- Onycholyse
- Onycholysis
- Onicólisis

Fig. 143 Onycholysis

- Onycholyse
- Onycholysis
- Onicólisis

Fig. 144 Leukonychia

- Leuconychie
- Leukonychie
- Leuconiquia

Fig. 145 Leukonychia

- Leuconychie
- Leukonychie
- Leuconiquia

Fig. 146 Herpetic whitlows

- Panarises herpétiques
- Umlauf bei Herpesinfektion
- Panadizos herpéticos

Fig. 147 Paronychia

- Paronychie
- Paronychie
- Oniquia periungueal

Fig. 148 Pyogenic granuloma

- Granulome pyogénique
- Pyogenes Granulom
- Granulome pyogénique

Fig. 149 Inclusion dermoid

- Dermoïde d'inclusion
- Dermoidzyste
- Dermoide de inclusión

Fig. 150 Hereditary haemorrhagic telangiectasia

- Maladie de Rendu-Osler
- Hereditäre hämorraghische Teleangiektasie
- Enfermedad de Rendu-Osler-Weber

Fig. 151 Osler's nodes

- Nodules d'Osler
- Osler-Knötchen
- Nudosidades de Osler

Fig. 152 Desquamation

- Desquamation
- Desquamation
- Descamación

Fig. 153 Desquamation

- Desquamation
- Desquamation
- Descamación

Fig. 154 Gouty tophi

- Tophus de la goutte
- Gichttophi
- Tofos en la gota

Fig. 155 Psoriatic arthropathy and nail dystrophy

- Rhumatisme psoriasique et dystrophie unguéale
- Psoriatische Arthropatchie und Nageldystrophie
- Psoriasis atrófico y distrofía ungular

Fig. 156 Dactylitis—psoriatic

- Dactylite—psoriasique
- Psoriatische Dactyliti
- Dactylitis—psoriática

Fig. 157 Dactylitis—infective

- Dactylite—infectieuse
- Infektiöse Dactylitis
- Dactylitis—infecciosa

Fig. 158 Melanin pigmentation

- Pigmentation de mélanine
- Melaninpigmentierung
- Pigmentación de melanina

Fig. 159 Melanin pigmentation

- Pigmentation de mélanine
- Melaninpigmentierung
- Pigmentación de melanina

Fig. 160 Vitiligo

- Leucodermie
- Vitiligo
- Vitíligo

Fig. 161 Steroid purpura

- Purpura stéroïde
- Steroidpurpura
- Púrpura esteroide

Fig. 162 Palmar erythema

- Érythéme des paumes
- Palmarerythem
- Eritema de las palmas

Fig. 163 Dermatomyositis

- Dermatomyosite
- Dermatomyositis
- Dermatomiositis

Fig. 164 Scleroderma

- Sclerodérmie
- Sklerodermie
- Escleroderma

Fig. 165 Scleroderma

- Sclerodérmie
- Sklerodermie
- Escleroderma

Fig. 166 Scleroderma

- Sclerodérmie
- Sklerodermie
- Escleroderma

Fig. 167 Dupuytren's contracture

- Maladie de Dupuytren
- Dupuytren-Kontraktur
- Contracción de Dupuytren

Fig. 168 Dupuytren's contracture

- Maladie de Dupuytren
- Dupuytren-Kontraktur
- Contracción de Dupuytren

Fig. 169 Dupuytren's contracture

- Maladie de Dupuytren
- Dupuytren-Kontraktur
- Contracción de Dupuytren

Fig. 170 Ulnar nerve palsy—claw hand

- Paralysie du nerf cubital—main en griffe

- Ulnarislähmung—Klauenhand

- Parálisis del nervio cubital—mano en garra

Fig. 171 Ulnar nerve palsy—claw hand

- Paralysie du nerf cubital—main en griffe

- Ulnarislähmung—Klauenhand

- Parálisis del nervio cubital—mano en garra

Fig. 172 Muscle wasting—first dorsal interosseus

- Atrophie musculaire—prèmier interosseux dorsal

- Muskelschwund—erster Interdigitalraum

- Artófia muscular—primer dorsal interóseo

Fig. 173 Rheumatoid arthritis—swan-neck deformities

- Polyarthrite chronique évolutive—déformités en col de cygne

- Rheumatoide Arthritis—Schwanenhalsdeformität

- Reumatismo articular crónico—deformidades de cuello de cisne

Fig. 174 Rheumatoid arthritis—boutonnière deformities

- Polyarthrite chronique évolutive—déformités boutonnière

- Rheumatoide Arthritis—Boutonnière Deformität

- Reumatismo articular crónico—deformidades boutonnière

Fig. 175 Rheumatoid arthritis—swan neck and Z-thumb deformities

- Polyarthrite chronique évolutive—déformités en col de cygne et pouce en Z

- Rheumatoide Arthritis—Schwanenhals-und 'Z-Daumen'-deformität

- Reumatismo articular crónico—deformidades de cuello de cisne y pulgar en forma de Z

Fig. 176 Rheumatoid arthritis—ulnar deviation

- Polyarthrite chronique évolutive—déviation cubitale

- Rheumatoide Arthritis—Ulnardeviation

- Reumatismo articular crónico—deviación cubital

Fig. 177 Rheumatoid arthritis—multiple deformities

- Polyarthrite chronique évolutive—déformités multiples

- Rheumatoide Arthritis—Multiple Verformungen

- Reumatismo articular crónico—deformidades múltiples

Fig. 178 Heberden's nodes

- Nodosités d'Heberden

- Heberden-Knoten

- Nodosidades de Heberden

Fig. 179 Heberden's and Bouchard's nodes

- Nodosités d'Heberden et Bouchard

- Heberden-und Bouchard-Knoten

- Nudosidades de Heberden y Bouchard

Fig. 180 Garrod's pads

- Nodosités de Garrod

- Garrod-Knötchen

- Nudosidades de Garrod

Fig. 181 Acromegaly

- Acromégalie

- Akromegalie

- Acromegalía

Fig. 182 Acromegalic and normal hands

- Mains acromegaliques et normales

- Hände bei Akromegalie und Hände eines Gesunden

- Manos acromegálicas y normales

Fig. 183 Cellulitis

- Cellulite

- Zellulitis

- Celulitis

Fig. 184 Cellulitis

- Cellulite

- Zellulitis

- Celulitis

Fig. 185 Track marks ('mainlining')

- Marques causées par des traces d'injection

- Injektionsstellen eines Drogensüchtigen ('Fixer')

- Marcas producidas por rastros de injección

Fig. 186 Lymphangitis

- Lymphangite

- Lymphangitis

- Linfangitis

Fig. 187 Lymphangitis

- Lymphangite
- Lymphangitis
- Linfangitis

Fig. 188 Olecranon bursa

- Burse olécrânienne
- Bursa olecrani
- Bolsa del olécrano

Fig. 189 Olecranon bursitis

- Bursite de l'olécrâne
- Bursitis olecrani
- Sinovitis bursal del olécrano

Fig. 190 Erythema nodosum

- Érythème noudeux
- Erythema nodosum
- Eritema nudoso

Fig. 191 Rheumatoid nodules

- Nodules rhumatoïdes
- Rheumaknötchen (Nodul rheumatici)
- Nódulos reumatoides

Fig. 192 Rheumatoid nodules

- Nodules rhumatoïdes
- Rheumaknötchen (Nodul rheumatici)
- Nódulos reumatoides

Fig. 193 Ganglion

- Ganglion
- Ganglion
- Ganglion

Fig. 194 Lipomata

- Lipomes
- Lipomata
- Lipoma

Fig. 195 Main d'accoucheur

- Main d'accoucheur
- Geburtshelferhand ('Pfötchenstellung')
- Mano obstétrica

Fig. 196 Pagetic forearm

- Maladie osseuse de Paget—avant-bras
- Unterarm bei Paget—Erkrankung
- Enfermedad de Paget—antebrazo

Fig. 197 Xanthomata

- Xanthomes
- Xanthome
- Xanthomas

Fig. 198 Xanthomata

- Xanthomes
- Xanthome
- Xanthomas

Fig. 199 Xanthomata

- Xanthomes
- Xanthome
- Xanthomas

Fig. 200 Lymphadenopathy

- Lymphadénopathie
- Lymphadenopathie
- Linfadenopatía

Fig. 201 Lymphadenopathy

- Lymphadénopathie
- Lymphadenopathie
- Linfadenopatía

Fig. 202 Acanthosis nigricans

- Acanthosis nigricans
- Acanthosis nigricans
- Acantosis nigracans

Fig. 203 Pseudoacanthosis

- Pseudoacanthosis
- Pseudoakanthose
- Seudoacantosis

Fig. 204 Gynaecomastia

- Gynécomastie
- Gynaekomastie
- Ginecomastia

Fig. 205 Galactorrhoea

- Galactorrhée
- Galaktorrhoe
- Galactorrea

Fig. 206 Breast abscess

- Abcés du sein
- Mammaabszess
- Abceso mamario

Fig. 207 Breast carcinoma

- Cancer du sein
- Mammakarzinom
- Cáncer de la mama

Fig. 208 Paget's disease of nipple

- Maladie de Paget du mamelon
- Paget Krebs der Mamille
- Enfermedad de Paget del pezón

Fig. 209 Breast carcinoma—nipple retraction

- Cancer du sein—mamelon rétracté
- Mammakarzinom—Retraktion der Brustwarze
- Cancer de la mama—pezón hundido

Fig. 210 Breast carcinoma—skin tethering

- Cancer du sein—lésions de la peau
- Mammakarzinom—Hautveränderungen
- Cancer de la mama—lesiones de la piel

Fig. 211 Breast carcinoma—peau d'orange

- Cancer du sein—peau d'orange
- Mammakarzinom—'Peau d'orange' (Orangenhaut)
- Cancer de la mama—edema cutáneo

Fig. 212 Post-irradiation telangiectases

- Télangiectases causées par irradiation
- Teleangiektasie nach Bestrahlung
- Telangiectasias post-irradiativas

Fig. 213 Hirsute female

- Femelle hirsute
- Hirsutismus bei einer Frau
- Mujer hirsuta

Fig. 214 Lanugo: anorexia nervosa

- Lanugo: anorexie mentale
- Lanugo: Anorexia nervosa
- Lanugo: anorexia mental

Fig. 215 Spina bifida occulta

- Spina bifida oculta
- Spina bifida occulta
- Espina bifida oculta

Fig. 216 Herpes zoster

- Zona
- Herpes zoster
- Herpes zóster

Fig. 217 Herpes zoster

- Zona
- Herpes zoster
- Herpes zóster

Fig. 218 Herpes zoster

- Zona
- Herpes zoster
- Herpes zóster

Fig. 219 Winged scapula

- Omoplate ailée
- Scapula alata
- Escápula alada

Fig. 220 Pectus carinatum

- Thorax en carène
- Kielbrust
- Pecho de pichón

Fig. 221 Pectus excavatum

- Thorax de cordonnier
- Trichterbrust
- Tórax de zapatero

Fig. 222 Scoliosis and café au lait patches

- Scoliose et plaques 'café au lait'

- Scoliose und 'café au lait' Flecke

- Escoliosis y manchas de 'café con leche'

Fig. 223 Kyphosis

- Cyphose

- Kyphose

- Cifosis

Fig. 224 Venous distension: superior vena cava obstruction

- Dilatation veineuse: obstruction de la veine cava supérieure

- Stauvenen: Obstruktion der Vena cava superior

- Dilatación de las venas: obstrucción de la vena cava superior

Fig. 225 Acne vulgaris

- Acné vulgaire

- Acne vulgaris

- Acne vulgar

Fig. 226 Umbilical psoriasis

- Psoriasis ombilicale

- Umbilikale Psoriasis

- Psoriasis umbilical

Fig. 227 Neurofibromatosis

- Neurofibromatose

- Neurofibromatose (v.Recklinghausen)

- Neurofibromastosis

Fig. 228 Abdominal distension with everted umbilicus

- Dilatation abdominale avec éversion ombilicale

- Auftreibung des Abdonem mit Nabelprolaps

- Dilatacion abdominal con eversión umbilical

Fig. 229 Pigmented scar: Addison's disease

- Cicatrice pigmentée: maladie d'Addison

- Hyperpigmentierte Narbe bei M. Addison

- Cicatriz pigmentada: enfermedad de Addison

Fig. 230 Gray-Turner's sign

- Signe de Gray-Turner

- Gray-Turner Zeichen

- Signo de Gray-Turner

Fig. 231 Cullen's sign

- Signe de Cullen

- Cullen Zeichen

- Signo de Cullen

Fig. 232 Striae: Cushing's syndrome

- Stries: syndrome de Cushing

- Striae: Cushing-Syndrom

- Estrías: síndrome de Cushing

Fig. 233 Striae gravidarum

- Vergetures de la grossesse

- Striae gravidarum

- Estrías astróficas

Fig. 234 Cushing's syndrome

- Syndrome de Cushing

- Cushing-Syndrom

- Síndrome de Cushing

Fig. 235 Simple obesity

- Obésité simple

- Fettsucht

- Obesidad simple

Fig. 236 Eunuchoid habitus: hypopituitarism

- Habitus eunuchoïde: hypopituitarisme

- Eunuchoider Habitus: Hypopituitarismus

- Hábito eunucoide: hipopituitarismo

Fig. 237 Inguinal lymphadenopathy

- Lymphadénopathie inguinale

- Inguinale Lymphadenopathie

- Linfadenopatía inguinal

Fig. 238 Tinea cruris

- Eczéma marginé de Hebra

- Tinea des unterschenkels

- Tina crural

Fig. 239 Hypogonadism

- Hypogonadisme

- Hypogonadismus

- Hipogonadismo

Fig. 240 Priapism

- Priapisme

- Priapismus

- Priapismo

Fig. 241 Penile warts

- Pénis verruqueux

- Verrucae penis

- Pene verrugoso

Fig. 242 Penile warts

- Pénis verruqueux

- Verrucae penis

- Pene verrugoso

Fig. 243 Primary chancre: syphilis

- Syphilis: chancre primaire

- Schanker: syphilitischer Primäraffekt

- Sífilis: chancro primitivo

Fig. 244 Herpes simplex

- Herpés

- Herpes simplex

- Herpes simple

Fig. 245 Psoriasis

- Psoriasis

- Psoriasis

- Psoriasis

Fig. 246 Lichen planus

- Lichen plan

- Lichen planus

- Liquen planus

Fig. 247 Circinate balanitis

- Balanite circiné

- Balanitis circinata

- Balanitis circinada

Fig. 248 Carcinoma

- Carcinome

- Karzinom

- Carcinoma

Fig. 249 Lichen sclerosus

- Lichen scléreux

- Lichen sclerosus

- Liquen escleroso

Fig. 250 Vulval ulcer

- Ulcère vulvaire

- Ulkus der Vulva

- Ulcera vulval

Fig. 251 Prolapsed haemorrhoids

- Prolapsus des hémorroïdes

- Prolabierte Hämorrhoiden

- Prolapso de hemorroides

Fig. 252 Thrombosed haemorrhoid

- Thrombose hémorroidale

- Thrombosierte Hämorrhoiden

- Trombosis en una emorroide

Legs and feet

Fig. 253 Onychogryphosis

- Onycogrypose

- Onychogryphosis

- Onicogriposis

Fig. 254 Subungual fibroma

- Fibrome subunguéal

- Subunguales Fibrom

- Fibroma subungular

Fig. 255 Clubbing

- Hippocratisme digital

- Trommelschlegelfinger

- Hipocratismo

Fig. 256 Vasculitic infarcts

- Calcification angéitique

- Vasculäre Infarkte

- Infartos calcáreos vasculiticos

Fig. 257 Digital gangrene

- Gangrène digitale

- Fingergangrän

- Gangrena digital

Fig. 258 Digital gangrene

- Gangrène digitale
- Fingergangrän
- Gangrena digital

Fig. 259 Arterial gangrene

- Gangrène artérielle
- Arterielle Gangrän
- Gangrena arterial

Fig. 260 Arterial gangrene

- Gangrène artérielle
- Arterielle Gangrän
- Gangrena arterial

Fig. 261 Venous gangrene

- Gangrène veineuse
- Venöse Gangrän
- Gangrena venosa

Fig. 262 Venous gangrene

- Gangrène veineuse
- Venöse Gangrän
- Gangrena venosa

Fig. 263 Rheumatoid arthritis—metatarsophalangeal subluxations

- Rhumatisme chronique progressif—subluxations métatarsophalangiennes
- Rheumatoide Arthritis—metatarsophalangeale Subluxation
- Reumatismo articular crónico—subluxaciones metatarsofalángicas

Fig. 264 Acute gout

- Goutte aigue
- Akuter Gichtanfall
- Gota aguda

Fig. 265 Hallux valgus

- Orteil en équerre
- Hallux valgus
- Hallux valgus

Fig. 266 Lymphangitis

- Lymphangite
- Lymphangitis
- Linfangitis

Fig. 267 Cellulitis

- Cellulite
- Zellulitis
- Celulitis

Fig. 268 Cellulitis—acute

- Cellulite—aigue
- Zellulitis—akut
- Celulitis—aguda

Fig. 269 Cellulitis—resolving

- Cellulite—en résolution
- Zellulitis—rekonvaleszent
- Celulitis—en trámites de resolución

Fig. 270 Erythema ab igne

- Érythème calorique
- Erythema ab igne
- Eritema calórico

Fig. 271 Varicose veins

- Varice
- Varizen
- Varices

Fig. 272 Varicose ulcer

- Ulcère variqueux
- Ulcus varicosum
- Ulcera varicosa

Fig. 273 Varicose ulcer

- Ulcére variqueux
- Ulcus varicosum
- Ulcera varicosa

Fig. 274 Vasculitic ulceration

- Ulcération angéitique
- Ulcus bei Vasculitis
- Ulceratión vasculitica

Fig. 275 Necrobiosis lipoidica

- Nécrobiose lipoïdique
- Necrobiosis lipoidica
- Necrobiosis lipoidea

Fig. 276 Trophic ulceration

- Ulcération trophique
- Ulcus trophicum
- Ulceración trófica

Fig. 277 Pitting oedema

- Oedème mou
- Vernarbendes Ödem
- Edema depresible

Fig. 278 Lymphoedema

- Lymphoedème
- Lymphödem
- Linfedema

Fig. 279 Lymphoedema

- Lymphoedème
- Lymphödem
- Linfedema

Fig. 280 Paget's disease

- Maladie osseuse de Paget
- M. Paget
- Enfermedad de Paget

Fig. 281 Paget's disease

- Maladie osseuse de Paget
- M. Paget
- Enfermedad de Paget

Fig. 282 Pretibial myxoedema

- Myxoedème pretibial
- Prätibiales Myxödem
- Mixedema pretibial

Fig. 283 Pretibial myxoedema

- Myxoedème pretibial
- Prätibiales Myxödem
- Mixedema pretibial

Fig. 284 Prepatellar bursa

- Burse prépatellaire
- Bursa praepatellaris
- Bolsa prerotular

Fig. 285 Prepatellar bursitis

- Bursite prépatellaire
- Bursitis praepatellaris
- Bursitis prerotular

Fig. 286 Erythema nodosum

- Érythème noueux
- Erythema nodosum
- Eritema nudoso

Fig. 287 Erythema nodosum

- Érythème noueux
- Erythema nodosum
- Eritema nudoso

Fig. 288 Muscle wasting—cachexia

- Atrophie musculaire—cachexie
- Muskelschwund—Kachexie
- Atrófia muscular—caquexia

Fig. 289 Muscle wasting—neuropathic

- Atrophie musculaire—neuropathique
- Muskelschwund—Neuropathie
- Atrófia muscular—neuropática

Fig. 290 Muscular dystrophy—pseudohypertrophy

- Paralysie musculaire—pseudohypertrophique
- Muskeldystrophie—Pseudohypertrophie
- Distrofia muscular—seudohipertrófica

Fig. 291 Muscular dystrophy—pseudohypertrophy

- Paralysie musculaire—pseudohypertrophique
- Muskeldystrophie—Pseudohypertrophie
- Distrofia muscular—seudohipertrófica

Fig. 292 Xanthomata

- Xanthomes
- Xanthome
- Xantomas

Fig. 293 Xanthomata

- Xanthomes
- Xanthome
- Xantomas

Fig. 294 Lipohypertrophy

- Lipohypertrophie
- Lipohypertrophie
- Lipohypertrofia

Fig. 295 Lipohypertrophy

- Lipohypertrophie
- Lipohypertrophie
- Lipohypertrofia

Fig. 296 Lipoatrophy

- Lipoatrophie
- Lipoatrophie
- Lipoatrofia

Fig. 297 Decubitus ulcers (pressure sores)

- Escarres (plaies de pression)

- Dekubitus (Druckpunkte)

- Ulcera por decúbito (llagas de presión)

Fig. 298 Decubitus ulcers (pressure sores)

- Escarres (plaies de pression)

- Dekubitus (Druckpunkte)

- Ulcera por decúbito (llagas de presión)

Skin

Fig. 299 Urticarial rash

- Éruption urticaire

- Urtikaria

- Erupción urticaria

Fig. 300 Macular rash

- Éruption maculaire

- Makula

- Erupción macular

Fig. 301 Papular rash

- Éruption papuleuse

- Papula

- Erupción papular

Fig. 302 Pustular rash

- Éruption varicelliforme de Kaposi

- Pustel

- Erupción variceliforme de Kaposi

Fig. 303 Vesicle

- Vésicule

- Bläschen

- Vesícula

Fig. 304 Vesicles

- Vésicules
- Bläschen
- Vesículas

Fig. 305 Bulla

- Ampoule
- Blase
- Ampolla

Fig. 306 Bulla

- Ampoule
- Blase
- Ampolla

Fig. 307 Purpura—vasculitic

- Purpura—myélopathique
- Purpura—Vasculitis
- Púrpura—reumática

Fig. 308 Purpura—thrombocytopenic

- Purpura—thrombopénique
- Purpura—Thrombozytopenie
- Púrpura—trombocitopénica

Fig. 309 Purpura—senile

- Purpura—sénile
- Purpura—senilis
- Púrpura—seníl

Fig. 310 Bruising

- Contusion
- Quetschung
- Contusiones

Fig. 311 Target lesions

- Lésions par irradiation
- Erythema multiforme
- Lesiones por irradiación

Fig. 312 Erythema marginatum

- Érythème marginé
- Erythema marginatum
- Eritema marginado

Fig. 313 Pigmented naevi

- Naevi pigmentaires
- Pigmentierte Nävi
- Nevos pigmentarios

Fig. 314 Café au lait patch

- Plaque café au lait
- Café au lait Flecke
- Mancha café con leche

Fig. 315 Comedones

- Comédons
- Comedones (Mitesser)
- Comedones

Fig. 316 Campbell de Morgan spots

- Taches de de Morgan
- Campbell de Morgan Flecke
- Manchas de de Morgan

Fig. 317 Spider naevi

- Angiomes stellaires
- Spider naevi
- Angiomas estelares

Fig. 318 Spider naevus

- Angiome stellaire
- Spider naevus
- Angioma estelar

Fig. 319 Spider naevus—blanching on pressure

- Angiome stellaire—blanchissement sous pression
- Spider naevus—Abblassung bei Druckeinwirkung
- Angioma estelar—palidecimiento bajo presión

Fig. 320 Dermographism

- Dermatographie
- Dermographismus
- Dermografismo

Fig. 321 Dermographism

- Dermatographie
- Dermographismus
- Dermografismo

Fig. 322 Ichthyosis

- Ichtyose
- Ichthyosis
- Ictiosis

Fig. 323 Ichthyosis

- Ichtyose
- Ichthyosis
- Ictiosis

Fig. 324 Atopic eczema

- Eczéma atopique

- Endogenes Ekzem (Eczema atopicum)

- Eczema atópico

Fig. 325 Atopic eczema

- Eczéma atopique

- Endogenes Ekzem (Eczema atopicum)

- Eczema atópico

Fig. 326 Atopic eczema

- Eczéma atopique

- Endogenes Ekzem (Eczema atopicum)

- Eczema atópico

Fig. 327 Dermatitis artefacta (self-mutilation)

- Dermatite artificielle (mutilation de soi-même)

- Dermatitis artefacta (Autoaggression)

- Dermatitis artificial (automutilación)

Fig. 328 Dermatitis artefacta (self-mutilation)

- Dermatite artificielle (mutilation de soi-même)

- Dermatitis artefacta (Autoaggression)

- Dermatitis artificial (automutilación)

Fig. 329 Dermatitis artefacta (cigarette burns)

- Dermatite artificielle (brûlures de cigarette)

- Dermatitis artefacta (Zigarettenbrandmal)

- Dermatitis artificial (quemaduras de cigarillo)

Fig. 330 Psoriasis

- Psoriasis

- Psoriasis

- Psoriasis

Fig. 331 Psoriasis

- Psoriasis

- Psoriasis

- Psoriasis

Fig. 332 Psoriasis

- Psoriasis

- Psoriasis

- Psoriasis

Fig. 333 Psoriasis

- Psoriasis
- Psoriasis
- Psoriasis

Fig. 334 Psoriasis

- Psoriasis
- Psoriasis
- Psoriasis

Fig. 335 Psoriasis

- Psoriasis
- Psoriasis
- Psoriasis

Fig. 336 Pityriasis versicolor

- Pityriasis versicolor
- Pityriasis versicolor
- Pityriasis versicolor

Fig. 337 Lichen planus

- Lichen planus
- Lichen planus
- Liquen planus

Fig. 338 Skin tags

- Molluscum pendulum
- Acrochordon
- Molusco péndulo

Fig. 339 Molluscum contagiosum

- Molluscum contagiosum
- Molluscum contagiosum
- Molusco contagioso

Fig. 340 Molluscum contagiosum

- Molluscum contagiosum
- Molluscum contagiosum
- Molusco contagioso

Fig. 341 Keloid scar

- Cicatrice cheloïdienne
- Keloid
- Cicatriz queloide

Fig. 342 Keloid scar

- Cicatrice cheloïdienne
- Keloid
- Cicatriz queloide

Fig. 343 Hypertrophic scar

- Cicatrice hypertrophique

- Hypertrophische Narbe

- Cicatriz hipertrófica

Fig. 344 Keratoacanthoma

- Hyperplasie pseudo-épithéliomateuse de la peau

- Keratoakanthom

- Seudoepitelioma espinocelular

Fig. 345 Basal cell carcinoma (rodent ulcer)

- Epitélioma basocellulaire (ulcus rodens)

- Basalzellkarzinom (Ulcus rodens)

- Carcinoma basocelular (ulcus rodens)

Fig. 346 Giant hairy naevus

- Naevus pileux géant

- Großer Naevus pilosus

- Nevo piloso gigante

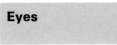

Eyes

Fig. 347 Cataract—black pupillary reflex

- Cataracte—réflexe pupillaire noir

- Katarakt—schwarzer Pupillenreflex

- Catarata—reflejo pupilar negro

Fig. 348 Cataract—white pupillary reflex

- Cataracte—réflexe pupillaire blanc

- Katarakt—weißer Pupillenreflex

- Catarata—reflejo pupilar blanco

Fig. 349 Cortical cataract

- Cataracte corticale

- Kataracta corticalis

- Catarata cortical

Fig. 350 Stellate cataract

- Cataracte étoilée

- Cataracta stellata

- Catarata cortical (estrellada)

Fig. 351 Intraocular lens implant

- Implant intraoculaire du cristallin
- Intraoculäres Linsenimplantat
- Injerto intraocular del cristalino

Fig. 352 Dislocated lens

- Luxation du cristallin
- Dislozierte Linse
- Luxación del cristalino

Fig. 353 Coloboma of iris

- Colobome de l'iris
- Coloboma iridis
- Coloboma del iris

Fig. 354 Irregular pupil: iritis

- Pupille irréguliére: iritis
- Unregelmäßige Pupille: Iritis
- Pupila desigual: iritis

Fig. 355 Nerve-fibre layer (flame) haemorrhage

- Hémorragie de la couche des fibres nerveuses
- Flammenförmige Blutung in der Nervenfaserschicht
- Hemorragia de la capa de fibras nerviosas

Fig. 356 Intraretinal (blot) haemorrhage

- Hémorragie intrarétinienne
- Intraretinale (Fleck-) Blutung
- Hemorragia intraretiniana

Fig. 357 Preretinal (subhyaloid) haemorrhage

- Hémorragie prérétinienne (subhyaloïde)
- Präretinale (subhyaloide) Blutung
- Hemorragia preretiniana (subhialoide)

Fig. 358 Subretinal haemorrhage

- Hémorragie subrétinienne
- Subretinale Blutung
- Hemorragia subretiniana

Fig. 359 Hard exudates

- Exudats rétiniens (durs)
- Harte Exsudate
- Exudados de la retina (duros)

Fig. 360 Hard exudates

- Exudats rétiniens (durs)
- Harte Exsudate
- Exudados de la retina (duros)

Fig. 361 Cotton wool spots (soft exudates)

● Exudats rétiniens (mous)

● Cotton-wool-Herde (weiche, wolkige Exsudate)

● Exudados de la retina (blandos)

Fig. 362 Drusen

● Drusen

● Drusen (Dalen–Körperchen)

● Gránulos

Fig. 363 Hypertensive retinopathy—arteriovenous changes

● Rétinopathie hypertensive—altérations arterio-veineuses

● Retinopathie bei Hypertension—arteriovenöse Veränderungen

● Retinopatía hipertensiva—cambios arteriovenosos

Fig. 364 Hypertensive retinopathy—arteriovenous changes

● Rétinopathie hypertensive—altérations arterio-veineuses

● Retinopathie bei Hypertension—arteriovenöse Veränderungen

● Retinopatía hipertensiva—cambios arteriovenosos

Fig. 365 Hypertensive retinopathy—accelerated hypertension

● Rétinopathie hypertensive—hypertension accélérée

● Retinopathie bei akzelerierter Hypertension

● Retinopatía hipertensiva—hipertensión acelerada

Fig. 366 Hypertensive retinopathy—accelerated hypertension

● Rétinopathie hypertensive—hypertension accélérée

● Retinopathie bei akzelerierter Hypertension

● Retinopatía hipertensiva—hipertensión acelerada

Fig. 367 Background diabetic retinopathy—minimal

● Rétinopathie diabétique générale—minimale

● Augenhintergrund bei minimaler Retinopathia diabetica

● Retinopatía diabética general—mínima

Fig. 368 Background diabetic retinopathy—mild

● Rétinopathie diabétique générale—benigne

● Augenhintergrund bei leichter Retinopathia diabetica

● Retinopatía diabética general—benigna

Fig. 369 Background diabetic retinopathy—moderate

- Rétinopathie diabétique générale—modérée

- Augenhintergrund bei mäsiger Retinopathia diabetica

- Retinopatía diabética general—moderada

Fig. 370 Diabetic maculopathy

- Maculopathie diabétique

- Diabetische Makulopathie

- Maculopatía diabética

Fig. 371 Background diabetic retinopathy—'dots' and small 'blots'

- Rétinopathie diabétique générale—points et petites taches

- Augenhintergrund bei Retinopathia diabetica—Punktblutungen und kleine Blutungsherde

- Retinopatía diabética general—puntos y pequeñas manchas

Fig. 372 Background diabetic retinopathy—red-free (green) illumination

- Rétinopathie diabétique générale—sous lumière pas-rouge (lumière verte)

- Augenhintergrund bei Retinopathia diabetica—grüne Beluchtung

- Retinopatía diabética general—bajo luz no roja (luz verde)

Fig. 373 Preproliferative diabetic retinopathy—cotton wool spots

- Rétinopathie diabétique préproliférative—exudats mous

- Präproliferative Retinopathia diabetica—cotton-wool-Herde

- Retinopatía diabética general—exudados blandos

Fig. 374 Preproliferative diabetic retinopathy—large blot haemorrhages

- Rétinopathie diabétique préproliférative—taches hémorragiques

- Präproliferative Retinopathia diabetica—großflächige Blutungsherde

- Retinopatía diabética general—manchas hemorrágicas

Fig. 375 Preproliferative diabetic retinopathy—beaded major vein

- Rétinopathie diabétique préproliférative—veine majeure perlée

- Präproliferative Retinopathia diabetica—Perlschnurartige Veränderungen einer Hauptvene

- Retinopatía diabética preproliferativa—vena mayor granulada

Fig. 376 Preproliferative diabetic retinopathy—venous loop (omega loop)

- Rétinopathie diabétique préproliférative—boucle veineuse (boucle oméga)

- Präproliferative Retinopathia diabetica—venöse Schleife (Omegaschleife)

- Retinopatía diabética preproliferativa—lazo venoso (lazo omega)

Fig. 377 Preproliferative diabetic retinopathy—ghost vessel

- Rétinopathie diabétique préproliférative—vaisseaux fantômes

- Präproliferative Retinopathia diabetica—'Schattengefäß'

- Retinopatía diabética preproliferativa—vaso fantasma

Fig. 378 Preproliferative diabetic retinopathy—preretinal (subhyaloid) haemorrhage

- Rétinopathie diabétique préproliférative—hémorragie prérétinale

- Präproliferative Retinopathia diabetica—präretinale (subhyoidale) Blutung

- Retinopatía diabética preproliferativa—hemorragia preretiniana

Fig. 379 Proliferative diabetic retinopathy—disc new vessels

- Rétinopathie diabétique proliférative—vaisseaux de disque nouveaux

- Proliferative Retinopathia diabetica—Gefäßneubildung an der Papille

- Retinopatía diabética proliferativa—vasos de disco recién formados

Fig. 380 Proliferative diabetic retinopathy—disc new vessels

- Rétinopathie diabétique proliférative—vaisseaux de disque nouveaux

- Proliferative Retinopathia diabetica—Gefäßneubildung an der Papille

- Retinopatía diabética proliferativa—vasos de disco recién formados

Fig. 381 Proliferative diabetic retinopathy—peripheral new vessels

- Rétinopathie diabétique proliférative—vaisseaux périphériques nouveaux

- Proliferative Retinopathia diabetica—periphere Gefäßneubildungen

- Retinopatía diabética proliferativa—vasos periféricos recién formados

Fig. 382 Proliferative diabetic retinopathy—fresh laser burns

- Rétinopathie diabétique proliférative—brûlures de laser récentes

- Proliferative Retinopathia diabetica—Zustand nach frischer Laserkoagulation

- Retinopatía diabética proliferativa—quemaduras de laser recientes

Fig. 383 Central retinal vein occlusion

- Occlusion de la veine centrale de la rétine

- Verschluß der Vena centralis retinae

- Oclusión de la vena central de la retina

Fig. 384 Branch retinal vein occlusion

- Occlusion d'une branche de la veine centrale de la rétine

  Verschluß eines Astes der Vena centralis retinae

- Oclusión de una rama de la vena central de la retina

Fig. 385 Central retinal artery occlusion

- Occlusion de l'artère centrale de la rétine

- Verschlußder Arteria centralis retinae

- Oclusión de la arteria central de la retina

Fig. 386 Branch retinal artery occlusion

- Occlusion d'une branche de l'artère centrale de la rétine

- Verschluß eines Astes der Arteria centralis retinae

- Oclusión de una rama de la arteria central de la retina

Fig. 387 Senile macular degeneration—drusen

- Dégénérescence maculaire sénile—drusen

- Senile Makuladegenaration—Drusen

- Degeneración macular seníl—gránulos

Fig. 388 Senile macular degeneration—atrophic ('dry')

- Dégénérescence maculaire sénile—atrophique ('sèche')

- Senile Makuladegenaration—Atrophie ('trocken')

- Degeneración macular seníl—atrófica ('seca')

Fig. 389 Senile macular degeneration—disciform ('wet')

- Dégénérescence maculaire sénile—disciforme ('humide')

- Senile scheibenförmige Makuladegenaration (Exsudate)

- Degeneración macular seníl—discoidea ('húmeda')

Fig. 390 Senile macular degeneration—disciform scare

- Dégénérescence maculaire sénile—cicatrice disciforme

- Senile scheibenförmige Makuladegenaration—Vernarbung

- Degeneración macular seníl—cicatriz discoidea

Fig. 391 Myelinated nerve fibres

- Fibres nerveuses myélinisées

- Myelin—Nervenfaser

- Fibras nerviosas mielinizadas

Fig. 392 Myopic disc

- Disque myopique

- Papille bei Kurzsichtigkeit

- Disco miopico

Fig. 393 Swollen disc—papilloedema

- Discite—oedème papillaire

- Geschwollener Discus nervi optici—Papillenödem

- Discitis—edema papilar

Fig. 394 Swollen disc—papillitis

- Discite—papillite

- Geschwollener Discus nervi optici—Papillitis

- Discitis—papilitis

Fig. 395 Normal optic disc cup

- Excavation normale du disque optique

- Normale excavatio disci

- Excavación del disco óptico normal

Fig. 396 Suspicious disc cupping

- Excavation suspecte du disque optique

- Verdächtige excavatio disci

- Excavación del disco óptico sospechosa

Fig. 397 Pathological disc cupping

- Excavation pathologique du disque optique
- Pathologische excavatio disci
- Excavación del disco óptico patológica

Fig. 398 Optic atrophy

- Atrophie optique
- Optikusatrophie
- Atrofia optica

Fig. 399 Retinitis pigmentosa

- Rétinite pigmentaire
- Retinitis pigmentosa
- Retinitis pigmentaria

Fig. 400 Angioid streaks

- Stries angioïdes de Knapp
- Angioide Netzhautstreifen
- Etrías angioides de la retina

Fig. 401 Toxoplasma choroiditis

- Choroïdite toxoplasmatique
- Choroiditis bei Toxoplasmose
- Coroiditis toxoplásmica

Fig. 402 Choroidal tumour

- Tumeur choroïdal
- Choroidtumor
- Tumor coroideo

Index